TOUR AOTEAROA

A GONZO CYCLING GUIDE

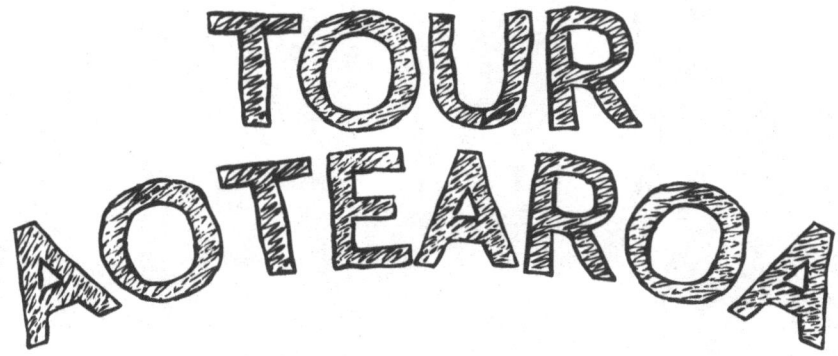

DUNCAN COUTTS

Published 2025
by Duncan Coutts

ISBN 978-0-473-74331-4 (International Edition)

© Copyright Duncan Coutts 2025

All rights reserved.

Except for the purpose of fair reviewing, no part of this publication may be reproduced or transmitted in any form or by any means, electronic or mechanical, including photocopying, recording or any information storage and retrieval system, without prior written permission from the publisher.

Cover illustration by Matt Ineson

Designed and distributed in New Zealand by CopyPress, Nelson, New Zealand.
www.copypress.co.nz

Contents

Epigraph vii

Foreword viii

Part One **Constant Companions**

Cape Reinga to Ahipara 3

Ahipara to Opononi 18

Opononi to Dargaville 25

Dargaville to Poutu Point 32

Helensville to Auckland City 40

Auckland 41

Auckland to Miranda Hot Springs 43

Miranda Hot Springs to Te Aroha 49

Te Aroha to Arapuni 59

Arapuni to Pureora 71

Timber Trail to Taumaranui 78

Part Two **The Little Things**

Taumaranui 89

Taumaranui to Whakahoro 94

Whakahoro to Pipiriki 97

Pipiriki to Whanganui 103

Whanganui to Rangiwahia 109

Rangiwahia to Pahiatua 125

Pahiatua to Martinborough 135

Martinborough 145

Part Three **Downhill, or Uphill – or Sometimes Both**

Martinborough to Wellington 149

Wellington to Pelorus Bridge 157

Pelorus Bridge to Wakefield 164

Wakefield to Murchison 171

Murchison to Reefton 181

Reefton 186

Reefton to Ikamatua 187

Ikamatua to Kumara 198

Kumara to Ross 205

Ross to Fox 210

Fox to Haast 216

Haast to Makarora 225

Makarora to Wanaka 228

Wanaka to Queenstown 231

Queenstown to Mossburn 235

Mossburn to Bluff 242

Thanks 252

Epigraph

Jonathan Kennett: co-creator of Tour Aotearoa – from an article in North and South magazine

To enter, participants make a $100 donation to a charity of their choice and pay to offset the carbon emissions they generate travelling to the start line in Cape Reinga and home from the finish in Bluff. Aside from that, it's all on the riders. After that initial flurry of interest in 2014, Kennett worried that he may have oversold how fun the experience would be. To discourage any inexperienced riders, he tried some anti-marketing. He posted a Shackleton-esque warning on Facebook: "You can expect to ride through horrible storms, suffer festering boils, crash and hurt yourself ... HONESTLY, I wouldn't enter if I were you." It didn't work. "That was like fodder to these guys," Kennett says. Two hundred and fifty people rode the first Tour Aotearoa in 2016.

Foreword

The TA (Tour Aotearoa) is a bicycle trail running the length of New Zealand but with kinks in it. The result: 3000 kilometres of trail that is in your backyard. Many Kiwis see some of it, dabble with bits of it. Few go the whole hog.

For someone like Duncan Coutts to even attempt Tour Aotearoa is pure madness. But sometimes a little madness can take a person a long way. In this case, a very, very long way.

This irreverent and at times insightful account of bikepacking the length of New Zealand is a unique mixture of fun, humour and, in a strange way, inspiration.

If Duncan and Homer can do it, anyone can!

I'm so glad you made it Duncan. Congratulations!

Pedal on!

Jonathan, the man of few words.

Jonathan Kennett: co-creator of Tour Aotearoa

PART ONE

Constant Companions

Cape Reinga to Ahipara

16km seal, 3km gravel, 84km beach

I struggled out of my tent. *My God, I should have tried that tent out before I signed up for this. It's like a child's plaything.* And the mattress was like sleeping on my high-school chemistry teacher. All bones, elbows and chalk dust. So narrow. You didn't roll over, you rolled off. Bloody hell, and this trip was going to be … how long?

Tapotupotu Bay and campsite were listed by DOC as being only a five-minute drive from Cape Reinga. Or, three hours' walking by track. That should tell you how steep the climb was.

'Dulp,' I coughed, slapping my head.

'Doh,' agreed Homer, not moving a millimetre. Homer was a seven-centimetre acrylic figurine, mounted on the stem of my touring bike. He couldn't really talk but I could hear him. Loud and clear. He was Homer Simpson after all. I mostly liked to cycle alone but I figured it could be good to have someone along to offer encouragement and advice. Homer was the man.

Headlamps flashed through thin nylon tents. It was somewhere between 5 and 6am. What time was sunrise? I could see other riders' shapes through the dark: wildly silhouetted wrestling bobcats and bears. In reality, they were just trying to reach their feet to put their socks on.

Must be a yoga name for this move, I reckoned. *Downward deformed dog.*

Today's beautiful weather forecast provided hope that the strong wind of yesterday wouldn't make another appearance. The TA, two years before, had featured a strong south westerly. TA riders took 11 hours to get halfway down 90 Mile Beach. It became a two-day forced ride. With a tailwind, it could be done in just three hours.

The more exclusive TA riders had shuttle vans and trailers to make the climb out of Tapotupotu Bay to get to the carpark at Cape Reinga. This was the official starting point: the gun was due to go off at 8am.

The mugs, the few of us who were riding up from the bay, packed our tents and sleeping gear. Headlamps flickered about madly. I was one of the last to leave – I was a little short on prep. And what did my footy coach used to say? *Piss Poor Preparation made for Piss Poor Performance.* Or was it something about potatoes? Anyway, I needed to get going; this was the first day and I had to at least look like I was ready.

The climb out of Tapotupotu Bay was steep and gravel. The deeper loams could catch an unwary wheel, pitch the cyclist face first to the ground. A gravel rashed chin would not be a good look to start the tour. Bottom gear was engaged – try not to let the heartrate rocket; it wasn't even sunup. I groaned deeply and considered walking. Walking the first 50 metres of the journey.

'Not on my watch,' said Homer.

Forty-five minutes later I panted my way into the Cape Reinga carpark. The place was chocka. Spandex and fluro milling about like a bad 80s dance party. I pushed my bike through to the back of the crowd. I couldn't help but notice the machinery – the bicycles. More gravel bikes than I expected. And a lot fewer gear bags on bikes than I expected.

Later that day I would find out why. Clever punters had left their gear at the Ahipara Campground and arrived at the cape with just a bare bike and a banana.

'Homer, preparation,' I muttered.

'You'll be fine,' replied Homer. 'Besides, bags act as sails and you'll be pushed by the wind all the way down the beach. Sweet sailing weather, me old chum.'

'Mate, there's no you. It's us.'

'Whaddaya mean?'

'You're coming too.'

'Hey, wait a minute pal. I've done the hard yards getting you to this stage. My job is done.'

I chuckled. 'Yeah, well good luck leaving. Your feet are screwed to the handlebars.'

'What, wait a minute,' bellowed Homer. 'You'll never get away with this.'

I wandered away from Homer's frantic shouting to get a look at my opposition. Fellow adventurers, is what I actually meant. *This wasn't a race, remember. Like hell.* There was a buzz of testosterone hovering over the crowd. And the woman equivalent – was that oestrogen? I wasn't an expert on the subject of women's parts, what made them tick. But I could smell the amping of ready, steady, go juice.

> Pre-race diarrhea is a standard nightmare … there are a lot of good reasons for dropping out of a race, but bad bowels is not one of them. The idea is to come off the line with a belly full of beer and other cheap fuel that will burn itself off very quickly. Carbo-power. No meat. Protein burns too slow for these people. They want the starch. Their stomachs are churning like rat-bombs and their brains are full of fear.
>
> *Hunter S Thompson.*

The crowd was assembled in clusters – mostly clusters of two – mostly guys, but some with 2 guys and a gal. Grouped together in animated dayglo Lycra conversation. The majority sported some kind of fluro clothing. *The day you get me in fluro is the day you'll put me in the ground*, I reckoned. My father always said you could tell a man by the way he wore his bicycle clips. My father would have rolled over in his grave had he seen the outfits these roosters were wearing.

There was the odd single rider. By 'odd', I meant odd, as in: who would do this ride without a mate's shoulder to cry on?

On looking closer, I realised there were plenty of lone riders, but they were not alone at this stage. They had their wives or partners standing listlessly beside them – for support; to make sure they started. Wives trying to look positive and engaged in the leaving ceremony but secretly wishing their husbands would make the whole trip and give them a month's peaceful break.

People looked very fit. The Spandex accentuated that. I had Spandex chamois shorts on but they were hidden, well covered by my baggy camo surf shorts. 'Can't ride a mountain bike with Lycra on mate,' my brother-in-law Murray always told me. 'Lycra's for the road jockeys.'

But *everyone* here had Lycra clothing, I noted. I was surprised by the number of gravel bikes. Gravel bikes looked like road racing bikes but they were specifically designed for gravel. Flexible frames and dampers. Large wheels with fat knobby tyres to absorb bumps and give grip. Very light.

Most people had gone for mountain bikes but not many had suspension. Or if they did, it was only the forks and the rear-end was a hardtail. This reassured me somewhat. The name Surly was conspicuous on many bikes. I knew a little about these bikes – steel framed, made in the USA. Mounting points everywhere for racks and bags. Strong, unbreakable. The Rolls Royce of touring bikes – nothing speaks real deal quite as much as a Surly.

But a bit heavy, I thought, with quiet but uneasy satisfaction.

I was starting to feel a little out of my depth. I was standing in the paddling pool looking out at the big kids splashing around in the big pool.

'C'mon, mate,' I muttered, to myself. 'Concrete pills. You've got this.'

I caught my foot on the edge of the paddling pool as I stumbled back to my bike. On the way I couldn't help noticing a young fella in a full Lycra skinsuit, complete with hood. He was doing big overhead stretches by a gravel bike. A bike, I noted dryly, with not a bag on it.

A tannoy sounded, giving everyone assembled a heads-up to pick up their tracking devices and be ready to leave at 8am. *Whoops nearly forgot.* I had been given a tracker by a friend of a friend. One that had been used a couple of years earlier; it wasn't in new condition. A spring for the batteries kept jumping out but it saved renting one. I registered with the organiser and readied myself.

A kaumatua from the local iwi gave a blessing. Then the organiser, from Map Progress, stepped forward to get us started. I expected him to be armed with a shotgun or a starting pistol – something grand and befitting the occasion. At least a flare gun.

A noise, a soft murmuring began amongst the riders. It rose as the crowd pushed forward. I could see the organiser trying to form some words but no chance, he was swept aside. The tour was beginning – there was no stopping it now. With a grand roar we were rolling. The organiser, still valiantly trying to say 'Bon Voyage' or some other weak 'Off you go now', was buried by the cavalcade. The mad crusade had begun.

I started from the back of the pack; I never did like to get the holeshot – even when I was racing motorbikes. I liked to have a hare to chase. Often, the real reason was that my bike had malfunctioned – an ignition wire had broken, the carbs had a leak.

There was much whooping and yahooing from the riders.

I still had a small warm glow of righteousness left over from the 45-minute warmup climb I had done from the beach campsite. So what if I was cold now – there would be no shortcuts on my trip. I was doing the whole trip and nothing but the trip – *so help me God.*

People looked decidedly cheery and fit. That word again kept popping into my head: fit. Hey, I had prepared. A month's cycling of South Island mountain bike tracks had hardened me. Sure, it had been on an e-bike. But you still had to work spinning the legs and the rides weren't short.

The battery got down to its last bar sometimes. However, there was always a café at the end, for incentive. But that was modern life, wasn't it? There was *always* a café at the end.

The first hour was a rollercoaster of hills to the turnoff to the famous Te Paki Stream. Cyclists were everywhere. Some stopped to wait for friends to catch up. Some stopped to adjust gear that had come loose.

I noted with some sympathy a rider on the side of the road. His bike was being attended to by some helpers from a van: it had a broken chain.

'That could be me,' I panted.

'Son, not with our maintenance program,' quipped Homer.

'What maintenance program?' I wheezed. 'Hope and cable ties. And what's with the son stuff? There's going to be no father-son type gig on this ride.'

The Te Paki Stream was at the end of a 3km gravel road.

I was blowing a bit. I stopped at a shelter just short of the stream to put on the stove. A cup of tea and some porridge – start this trip as I meant to go on. I had a trusty Trangia spirits stove with me, like the one I'd used when I cycle-toured in Europe in the early 80's. In fact, it looked exactly like the one I had used. That would make it antique; like me.

The design hadn't changed at all since the Swedish firm introduced it in 1951. Look how good the cars were in 1951? The washing machines. The typewriters. Was the early 50's a fantastic era for design? I wasn't so sure.

I knew the simple workings of a Trangia. Unscrew the lid of the burner, pour the meths into the fuel unit – a little dab behind each ear for luck – then throw a match at it and run and dive into a trench. Or beneath some sort of cover. Something like a sheet of corrugated iron.

A cup of tea was the first thing I stumbled for each morning. This morning had been somewhat disrupted. However, I believed I could recover my ken.

The porridge came to the boil. I watched with enjoyment the riders filing past the shelter – waving to me before tentatively diving their bikes into the shallow Te Paki to ride its stream down to the sea.

I also noticed that no others were stopping at the breakfast stop – okay, it wasn't an official stop but it was the most obvious place for breakfast – to me. By the time I had cleaned and packed again, there was little in the way of bike traffic. In fact, there hadn't been another cyclist for a good, wee while.

No worries. It's not a race.

The Te Paki Stream was shallow and interspersed with sandbanks. Keeping an eye out for cycle tyre tracks meant I could spot the best lines on the firmest sand. This would become something of a spoor for me – others' tyre tracks: brilliant.

'There's madness to my method,' I chuckled.

'Madness, anyway,' chuckled Homer.

A tailwind pushed me along the Te Paki Stream. I smiled all the way. I stopped grinning when the tailwind turned to a sidewind, I was now on 90-Mile Beach.

The beach stretched further north to the top. 90-Mile Beach wasn't really 90 miles, it was only 55 miles long. It got the name because the European settlers knew their horses could do 30 miles in a day. The beach took them three days. They hadn't realised the sand slowed the horses down.

South was where my destiny lay.

The sand was hard enough to ride on but it was a couple of gears down from pavement. The high line looked to be the one most firm and I set off. I noted dryly the wind was now filling my left ear – a sidewind with a hint of head in it.

Twelve kilograms was a figure I had heard mentioned regarding how much weight on average a rider lost doing the TA. Doubtful, I thought – that's somewhere near 25 blocks of butter. Most of the cyclists I had seen would be reduced to the size of split pins if they lost that much weight.

I had left the training regime to Homer, for better or worse. Homer claimed he had experience – military training. The plan was to not over train but to build strength in the first week of the tour. And with the weight thing, to take on the camel theory: to go in slightly overweight and live off one's self. To use the body as a feed station. Food supplies were not always going to be easy to obtain so living off your own fat cells could be a stroke of genius.

Carbs, carbs, carbs were Homer's mantra. *Yeah, right. So was beer, beer, beer.*

The camel theory had always seemed a little dubious to me. Combining that, with the weight of my bike, (which looked to be a little heavier than others), I started doubting whether putting the campaign strategy in Homer's hands was a good idea. To be honest I had many doubts. But, at least Homer had a plan; I had to admit that.

A few hours went by and I could have sworn I was in a spin class with the screen showing an endless beach scene curving away into the distance. Except for that buffeting wind from the left – a spin class didn't have wind effects.

I tried to relax into the moment, let spin music fill my head – The Police for inspiration, then a bit of AC/DC to keep me pumped and moving. But that damned wind kept lifting my hands from the handlebars.

Cycling required rhythm. On a long gradual downhill you could hit the big gears and stretch out the body – the legs circling in fine big arcs. Sit the bum back on the seat and lengthen the spine – take a back stretch, work the kinks out of the lumbar. Stay in that groove, that rhythm.

On the flat, up the cadence and channel the body into an aero position. Come the hills and it was more of a mind game – how hard did you want to push it? Get up on the pedals to crest a rise or simply to feel a change of pace.

The important thing was to rotate those legs: to feed the rhythm – feel the feet pushing and pulling in sweet circles – not to let the legs slump into 'pedalling squares' as the pros called it, when inefficiency took over.

I squinted into the distance, seeking relief. There was no rhythm to be found in this seemingly endless grind – what with the gusting wind and the soft patches of sand, I was struggling big time. If this was live television the commentators would be gleefully describing how I had hit the wall, was 'pedalling squares.' I could hear them: *'Look at the weaving upper body. The body may be there, folks, but the mind has gone. He's now in the hurt house: a world of pain.'* All of the cycling clichés.

I had cycled in Whangārei, a few months earlier, with a chap I'd met at the local bike park. The fella was from Auckland and was up north on holiday. His wife had dropped him at the park and he was to meet her further north. This bloke was full of beans – an 'Energizer Bunny'. He had done the TA the year before and averaged 30kph down 90-Mile Beach. He said he had arrived at Ahipara and looked back up the beach: 'Mate, I couldn't see anyone'.

The experience was proving a little different for me. I was pedalling in the same gear, with the same body position and the same bum on seat position – locked in some kind of time continuum. There was no getting comfortable or becoming in-tune with this moment.

I tried sitting slightly to the left, then to the right, then forward, then more to the back – no relief.

The bicycle saddle would become a large topic of conversation during the first week of the TA. I had researched and gone with a saddle that had scored four out of five stars in the reviews, I had settled on a Fizik. The Movistar cycling team used Fizik; if it was good enough for the pros it was good enough for me. A pro cycling team did a couple of hundred kilometres in a day – you didn't hear them bleating about their sore bottoms.

It was all about the sit bones. The chafing that occurred over this part of the anatomy. I didn't even know I had sit bones. I thought you sat on your bum. *Wasn't that what that was for?* Otherwise, what was the point of carrying that mound of flesh around behind you? If it wasn't for sitting on, then what other application could it possibly be used for?

I shifted again on my fancy Fizik seat. Orr, it was uncomfortable. On a bicycle seat, I realised the ample bum was of no use. It just filled out your pants.

Turned out there's a couple of wee bones inside the bum that did the sitting on the bike seat. A layer of flesh covered those bones – round about the crease line on the bottom. This crease line would rub back and forwards with each rotation of the pedals.

A whole world of lubricating butt cream was revealed to me. There were tubs of Butt Butter, Squirrels Saddle Butter, Aussie Butt Cream. My favourite was Brazilian Bum Bum Cream. Or you could get it in a tube. Chamois Butter, Antifriction Cream, Sweet Cheeks. I was on the Chamois Butter – a large tube.

It's not a world I chatted to any friends about. Didn't confess I was on the bum juice; the butt cream. Perhaps a confessional was where to take the matter. 'Forgive me father for I have chafed.'

I had liberally and secretly swabbed myself with butt cream that morning after packing up my camp. The problem was that this left tell-tale white cream on my hands. *Everyone knows what I've just been doing.* I had tried to wipe it off on the ground. It was no use: the layer of thick cream was still there, but now covered with twigs and grass.

I seemed to be magnifying the problem. The butt cream was incredibly sticky – I guessed it had to be to adhere to a sweaty arse working back and forth for hour after hour. *Imagine that as a job description*, I thought. *Imagine saying: 'I'm a butt cream designer.'* Would make your mother proud – a difficult conversation when asked what her boy was doing for a job.

This was a conundrum – I needed to regularly use the product, but how to clean up afterwards? Carrying a rag was not an option: it would quickly become matted with butt cream, and possibly other unmentionables. I had tried rubbing my hands down the bark of a tree. This left me with twigs, grass and now bark, attached to my palms; a regular little potpourri. I had resignedly pulled on my cycling gloves over the mess.

Later I discovered the cream made a perfect zip lubricant for my panniers, which were often a little stuck – that was the place to wipe your hands: run the fingers up and down the zips.

Twenty kilometres down the beach and I was becoming well acquainted with my sit bones – my constant companions as they would come to be known. I tried adjusting myself again but there's not a lot of choice on a skinny piece of plastic covered by a layer of foam and vinyl.

I had plenty of time to contemplate the areas of suffering my body was going through. Same grinding pace in the same gear. Neck and shoulders stiffening. The endless summer scene hazed ahead. Sun searing the back of my neck while the relentless wind bore further into my left ear canal. The first day was always the hardest; everyone who knew anything always said that. After that you're away. *Yeah, right. If you survive the first day.*

No one would know if I snuck away into the dunes for a wee lie-down. Then ditch the bike and my gear. Change into civvies and thumb a ride from a returning beach fisherman – down the beach to Ahipara. To the fish and chip shop. Then a bus home. No one would know. No one would miss me. I was on my own. My own!

'I'm on my own!' I gasped.

'You've got me, buddy,' corrected Homer. 'You're doing fine.'

'You think?'

'Absolutely. I've seen grown men crying at less than this.'

I relaxed a little. 'Thanks, Homer. Maybe I am doing okay.'

'Well, no. I didn't exactly say that.'

'What do you mean?'

'We don't seem to be moving. Are we stuck in some quicksand or something?'

I was falling into a bad schtick, and it was then that I noticed a shape ahead in the distance. In the not-too-distant distance. It appeared stopped.

As I drew closer I realised it was a person – a bloke. Another cyclist – a TA'er? I cycled earnestly towards him. I got close – he didn't look like a TA'er. This fella wasn't wearing Lycra shorts. Oh no, he was sporting Hawaiian style surf shorts, topped by a Hawaiian style shirt – a button up shirt with collar. His feet weren't enclosed in cleated shoes or flats – the fancy name for mountain bike flat-soled shoes. He was wearing open-toed sandals – Roman sandals.

His bike had no panniers but sported a rear rack on which was strapped a large roll bag, which was sagging dangerously to one side, blown that way by the wind. On the bars was a small handlebar bag. The most glaring piece of luggage was the yellow PVC newspaper satchel thrown over his shoulder. I knew it was a paper delivery bag: 'The Herald' was stamped in the middle of each side.

I was enchanted. This could well be a man I could respect, I thought, as I drew closer. Due to his girth the rider was not as short as he first appeared. He had thick unruly hair and a matching beard. He looked a lot like John Belushi. JB for short.

JB was head down in his satchel which he had swung onto the frame bar in front of him. He had two sandwiches in his left hand and a can of creaming soda in the right.

'Oh hi,' gulped JB, a somewhat surprised look on his face. He hadn't heard my approach. Not surprising with the noise of the wind.

(Actually, it was more like, 'Ooof, haaa,' as JB's mouth was full of sandwich.)

'Gidday,' I greeted. 'Looks like you're having a picnic on the go.'

'Yes. Trying to lighten the load. I brought too much gear. Well too much food really.'

I noticed some crusts lying on the sand. JB's beard was strung with crumbs – salad clung to his moustache. Tomato and what appeared to be cheese had fastened on his collar. Further down his Hawaiian gastronomic palette was some egg salad – laid between two palm trees – a poultry hammock.

What kind of picnic is this? It's more like a feeding frenzy.

'You want a sandwich?' asked JB enthusiastically. 'A creaming soda?' He held up the can. 'They're a bit warm but they're certainly creamy.'

'No thanks. I'm still trying to digest my breakfast.' I wanted no part of this torrid banquet.

JB burped long and expansively. 'So, you must be the last one.'

'What do you mean, last one?'

'The last rider.' JB looked over my shoulder up the beach from whence we'd come. 'No one's come past me for ages. And believe me, plenty came past me.' He chuckled. 'Still, it's not a race, is it?'

'Umm no,' I agreed doubtfully. *It now felt like more of a race than ever.* JB didn't even look like he'd make the third 15. Yet here he was declaring *me* to be the last.

'I broke my chain only a few km's from the cape,' continued JB. 'So it hasn't been the best of starts.'

So that was this guy. The guy on the side of the road with the broken chain. He didn't have proper luggage. He had a paper boy's satchel bulging with food. He had Roman sandals on his feet, for Pete's sake. And he was ahead of me!

How slow am I?

Pretty slow confirmed Homer.

I shook my head and tried to rationalise this, the first day. Everyone said it was the toughest – no matter which direction the wind. Obviously this side wind was better than one on the nose. Many had stashed their gear at the Ahipara campsite, so were running light bikes. Most had not made the gruelling climb up from Tapotupotu Bay. Still, even this guy JB was ahead.

'We should team up,' enthused JB.

He seemed remarkably upbeat and positive. I had to admit this was highly commendable considering where we were coming in the field. If we were racehorses we would have been shot.

'Just for today, of course,' said JB, taking my pause in the conversation as hesitancy.

'No, no.' I answered. 'I mean, yes. Of course. Makes sense. Now which way are we headed? Any ideas?'

'Ha. I like a man with a sense of humour,' laughed JB.

I joined JB in the impromptu picnic. Not from JB's satchel but from my own bags – I too could do with lightening the load. I didn't have nearly as much in the way of food stocks as JB, but every ounce less would make the journey easier; we had to make the best of this day somehow.

Carbs, carbs, carbs: the porridge hadn't given me the boost I thought it would. I had gone into the TA with some information, some ideas, but little in the way of tested concepts. I did know that information only became knowledge when tested. The "testing" schedule had not fitted my timetable in the build-up to the TA. The Discovery Channel had documented the Tour de France riders' training regime and diets: they would eat pasta morning and night. Also, potatoes – carbohydrates was the formula.

I scoffed a potato salad, chased by a can of baked beans. *Carbs, carbs, carbs.*

For some obscure reason, in preparation for the tour, I had read T E Lawrence: Notes on Camel Journeys, which had been published in 1919. It somehow seemed apt to recall it for this day: JB and I were surely the donkeys/camels of the TA field.

Only she-camels were used for endurance racing. Riders often changed camels in the longer distance races : 'A race of this sort is a test of the man's endurance, rather than that of the camel'. Lawrence covered a race from Medina to Mecca, by the Rabegh Rd – 450km. The average speed was 11kph.

Another equally noble effort was that of Aissa, a Harb tribesman. He travelled from Zilfi, in Qasim, to Yenbo in three days and returned to Zilfi in four more. A total of seven days round trip and 1450km at an average of 209km a day. Aissa used four camels.

A Sherari camel was one of the finest breeds; the Surly bicycle was not even a twinkle in its inventor's eye in the early 1900's. A stripped racing camel could do close to 30kph for nearly two hours. A short burst could be a little quicker and a cantering camel could hit a little over 40kph.

This recall was completely of no use to me in this situation; and showed the depth of gully my state of mind had fallen into. You would think I could dredge up a snippet of something valuable but alas my thoughts often turned to foolishness at the most inopportune moments.

JB and I ground our frazzled bodies down the beach, our feet pulled back on the pedals, up, forward, down – clunked movements instead of nice fluid circles. There was no question about it, we were pedalling squares.

I felt my last remaining energy draining away: the further dose of carbs meant any remnants of power in my body were now being used to digest, instead of powering up the muscles.

JB and I rode into the Ahipara campground 10 hours after the start at Cape Reinga – three hours later than the next slowest riders that day. The other riders were showered, had eaten and were full of bonhomie. The cabins were of course all taken. JB took the last bunk bed in the dormitory. I set up my tent.

Ahipara to Opononi

65km seal, 22km gravel

'Always look on the bright side of life.' Music was filtering through the bathroom speakers.

I had taken on some canned curry the evening before. It had me on the toilet early. The sun was barely rising. Fred Dagg being played through the camp's bathroom speakers: 'Always look on the bright side of life.'

Oh the irony, I sighed. Still, it was a new day and there wouldn't be another ride along a beach on this trip. Well not intentionally. I hadn't slept badly, 5 out of 10 would be the score. Exhaustion was no surety of a good night's sleep; I had issues there.

At least today the group would be starting on an even footing. The other TA'ers would be carrying full kit like me. Ok, perhaps not quite as much kit as me. I did appear to have quite a bit. But I would watch closely and observe the habits of my fellow cyclists.

Head lamped riders clomped about in their cleated shoes and Spandex. I noted with quiet satisfaction that most weren't quite so cheery this morning – not natural early risers, such as myself. Porridge was brought to the boil and I set it aside while I sorted my gear in the tent. I broke down camp and surprisingly it all went together well. When the bags were packed there was no errant gear lying about.

Two cups of tea, a plate of porridge with bananas and I was ready for the day. There was no sign of JB but I figured my fellow back marker was the kind who slept late. No starting at the back for me today. No sir. I needed to show this tour and myself that I was made of sterner stuff. It was every dog for itself today.

I didn't have a perfect navigation system organised. In fact, navigation hadn't featured high on the preparation list. I was a great list maker though, so that had to count for something. There were lists on the fridge, in the garage and notes all over the inside of my car. Some people used their phones to keep an orderly list of 'to do's'. I kept lists on random bits of paper.

The TA organisers had put out two official guides for the tour: one for the North Island and one for the South Island. Nice sized booklets which could be slid into a pocket or stuffed down one's shorts, under the butt area – over the sit bones.

The guides featured an introduction on what to expect – the surfaces likely to be ridden over and an Environmental Care Code. The TA was divided into sections with a mileage given of what surface would be ridden on for that section and a graph to show how steep it was.

I hadn't read the guides, which was fortunate – *but not*. The graphs often resembled outlines of the world's great peaks. If I had, for instance, glanced at the Palmerston North to Pahiatua graph, I would have put a match to the guide and gone straight for the fridge.

I figured I would take each day as it came and use the guide accordingly. Some folk tore each day's ride out of the booklet and stuck it somewhere up front – usually on display on their handlebar bag.

There was a set of GPS coordinates which could be downloaded onto your phone or GPS device, if you were lucky enough to have such a thing. Or knew how to work one. I wasn't particularly tech savvy but I did have a phone mount on my bars and a rain cover for the phone. I knew how to pull up the Google map of NZ and zoom it in; the blue dot was me. I failed to realise the app was modelled on the user being in a car. I could pull out the TA guide whenever it was necessary. Besides I would be with other cyclists. There would always be one ahead in the distance; *the next target*.

'Wait a minute, this just isn't a race,' said Homer, as I swung a leg over the bike.

'You are dead right, little buddy,' I agreed.

'This is sport – life and death. Way more important. Let's go get 'em pal.'

I was not going to be drawn into that competitive mind set. *There was no level playing field out here.* Most riders had packed lean and there was little evidence of a tent, sleeping gear or cooking device. I had all of those. And more, much more.

Your average TA rider's kit was compact. A tail bag poking out behind the saddle, waggling endearingly from side to side. Inside it was likely to be some lightweight multi-use designer clothing. A triangular frame bag sat inside the frame but had limited capacity – just enough space for a laundry bag or a pair of Gucci loafers. A couple of pouches fitted to the top bar. They contained nuts and raisins, a massage voucher.

The handlebar bag was solely for electronics. Tablet, electronic notebook, backup hard drive, powerpack – *and perhaps a set of small but perfectly formed NASA engineers.*

The cyclists with these lean setups were staying in motels or cabins. These had mostly been pre-booked. There was talk of a rider who did last year's tour with just the clothes he wore and a credit card.

There was also talk of a rider who did the tour only eating pies. There was talk of a rider who did the whole thing in just eight days – 3000 km in eight days. There was a lot of talk.

Some keen riders began leaving before daylight. I quickly got myself together, had a quick last scan of the ground for any fallen objects and rose onto my saddle to pedal out into the brave new world.

My constant companions instantly awoke; so early to make an appearance. I hoped desperately the sit bones would behave today and just enjoy the ride. At the camp exit I looked desperately both ways for the cyclists who had just left. I spied a flickering red tail light and set off in pursuit. *Not race pursuit* mind, just a moderate tailing speed.

Broadwood General Store was the first shop of the tour. Exciting. There were several riders in varied levels of repose outside the store. Leaning on the wall or sitting on some benches. They looked at ease, like they did bike packing every day.

It wasn't quite the café I had envisioned when dreaming about the tour. There was coffee available sure, but it came from a machine with buttons marked coffee, tea, hot chocolate. Still, it was hot.

Where was the cabinet with fresh muffins, cheese scones and quiche? There was a pie warmer; Big Ben was back. I wasn't again going to get sucked into loading my gut with a brick of carbohydrate. I chose bananas and remembered I had a One Square Meal bar in my bag. OSM. Not, OMG. Or, SOS. Or, FOMO. Or, MILF. *When did milk get spelt with an F?*

Outside the store, I carefully studied what each rider was consuming while he or she attempted to appear chilled and cool, like they knew what they were doing. Some were eating bananas. A couple were well into pies. One was munching a handful of gingernut biscuits. Simon, a chap I had spoken with earlier, was drinking a litre of milk. Interesting. *Must study these alien creatures.* They were giving me no dietary clues at this stage as to how to best the day.

A tailwind sprung up as I broached a hill and got my first glance of the Hokianga Harbour. The upper reaches of the harbour were bound on both sides by the ubiquitous mangrove – the beloved or hated mangrove.

The wind strengthened and swept me along the road beside the harbour; today was God's apology for yesterday – 25kph and rising. Now this was how the tour was supposed to roll.

To celebrate I pulled into the Kohukohu General Store and ordered a vanilla milkshake – the first of many on this tour. Then it was a quick sprint to the car ferry for the 10-minute sailing to Rawene. Too easy.

I was one of a group today. We mingled and chatted. We rode together the curves and hillocks towards that day's destination, Opononi.

However, I couldn't help but notice that when the road opened up the crowd soon thinned.

There was a long and steep hill just before Opononi. It was here that I made a magical discovery. I discovered the gift of walking – walking the bicycle. Ahead I had spied a fellow TA'er walking his bike up a hill. *You couldn't walk. That would be cheating, wouldn't it?* It's a cycle tour. *But walking meant you would still be doing it under your own steam.* Besides, in bottom gear on my bike, with my limited gear cluster I was only doing 5kph. Walking would be 4kph. At worst 3.5. I could feel a sense of guilt. *But why?*

I looked behind – there was no one in sight. *Who would know? Isn't cycling cheating, anyway? Walking the length of NZ: now that is a noble endeavour. That's truly a grind. Walkers are the true warriors.*

I dismounted and started pushing my bike. My constant companions were instantly silenced. It felt fantastic. My legs rested the cycling muscles and engaged the walking ones.

'Hey buddy, what are you doing?' said Homer, fearfully waking from his reverie.

'I'm walking.' I let out a small chuckle. 'And it feels great.'

'Are you quitting?' Homer was still using the small voice.

'No. I'm resting while still moving forwards. Still following the trail.'

'Get back on that bike, NOW!' bellowed Homer. 'We will not be beaten. We did not become the most powerful nation in the world by giving in. We are still the greatest.'

I laughed. 'Umm, mate, I think you've misplaced your geographic arse for just a moment.'

'I won't forget this moment,' muttered Homer. 'Weakness.'

Opononi, home of the legend of Opo, the dolphin that adopted the harbour in front of the village as its home. Where it would frolic with tourists and Opononians in a gentle fashion – allowing them to hang onto its fin for joyrides.

Hmm, I thought, gazing out at the serene waters. (I bet it wasn't all beer and skittles for Opo. There was often bound to be some little shit nagging the hell out of him.)

Opononi, a town of baches and shacks, looked out over the harbour to massive sand dunes on the other side. The fishing was magnificent on the west coast, but you had to know your way around the dangerous bars at the entrance to the harbour. *Drunks everywhere.*

I hadn't fully appreciated the campground back at Ahipara. I'd been a stumbling, bumbling, TA tumbleweed as I had entered its grounds. Plus, it had been nearly dark. Later I would come to realise it was the best campground on the whole tour.

The Opononi campground setting was spectacular – it possibly had the best *view* of the campgrounds on the tour. It was a shame it had been let go – left to seed; unloved. Plus, it was $25 for a tent site: Ahipara was $20. Ahipara had a glorious lounge with Sky TV, with cricket on. That hadn't seemed a big deal at the time but it was huge. It also had a fully equipped kitchen with bells and whistles – hard to find bells and whistles.

Opononi on the other hand had a kitchen of sorts: some gas burners and two sinks – not a pot or a pan. It did have showers. Showers that were well passed their use-by date but the water was warm – well appreciated by a sweaty cyclist. And a laundry – which was also a welcome sight. The rotary clothesline outside was curious. I noticed that cycle shorts, bibs, socks and shirts were arranged in a perfect circle beneath it. Nothing was hanging on the lines. *Aha, very windy and no pegs.*

The only pegs I had were tent pegs. Confusing for those learning the English language. *These are called pegs. And these are called pegs.*

It was no mean feat getting the pup tent connected to the ground as the wind was up. Eventually I got the thing nailed down and headed to the pub.

Dinner that evening was at the magnificently rustic Opononi Hotel

– the scene of many a fishy tail and the occasional flying jug. I went for the lasagne; carbs were the call for the evening meal: not during the day.

Unfortunately they were out of lasagne so a beef burger and fries became the go to. Our table was beset by TA riders and tales were exchanged, although to be fair, it was only day two so there weren't many tales. And no one was yet brave enough to relive day one on the beach. That subject was off the menu, along with the lasagne.

I had a pint of pilsner to recharge as I was weary. All it did was make me feel woozy. That's not a good sign I thought, blearily. Usually a beer recharged me. I bumbled slowly back to the campground, imagining a luxurious king-sized bed and a goose down pillow. *Come on mate, harden up.*

Opononi to Dargaville

58 km seal, 28km gravel

Headlamps on as TA cyclists went through the routine of packing and stacking tents. There were only seven tents set up in the Opononi campground. Goodness knows where the other 83 riders who started with me were staying. I knew some were in cabins at the campground. Some may have ridden further yesterday. I supposed the others must be in hotels or holiday homes nearby. These and many other thoughts were going through my head as I lay on the narrow airbed decompressing it. Rolling it down to the size of a cigarette. *Hard to believe you could sleep on a cigarette. Snap out of it, mate. Time for action.* Tea, porridge and ride. I had a bottle cage strapped low on the bike frame, just up from the bottom bracket. I made an extra tea in a thermal cup and slid it into the cage – it would stay warm for another hour – another cuppa further down the road. It's the small things that kept you going.

Mmmmnnn tea, I thought. *Mmmmnn beer,* thought Homer.

My legs were sore but alright. They warmed up once they'd been ticking over for an hour. I did have sore nipples though, chafed by my flapping shirt. This was not an uncommon issue on the tour. Band-Aids were the cure: not so much fun removing them.

Northland, with its volcanic past, was made up of a series of hills – some short and violent. NZ lay on the boundary between two tectonic plates, hence all the action. The North Island had the distinction of having all three types of volcano: Caldera – Taupo, Rotorua and Okataina, Cone – Ruapehu and Ngaruhoe, Volcanic

Fields – Auckland. Some were still active; some were waiting. In fact, I was to find out that the North Island was tougher climbing than the South Island.

The elevation line on the graph in the TA guide began smoothly enough. Suddenly it went vertical as if the author had slipped with his pen. A 300-metre climb within five kilometres – only just rideable for me and that was in bottom gear – the 5kph gear. I considered briefly having a walk but it was the start of the day and I didn't want Homer to start in again.

The view from the top of the climb was glorious. The Hokianga Harbour in all its morning glory spread below. The trees on the point were bent horrifically towards the west. Either a nasty deformation or a testament to some spiteful easterlies.

The café at Waimamaku was closed; no tourists. Huge kauri stumps littered a paddock in Waimamaku – ancient stumps pulled from the swamps. Then turned into furniture and crafts to be sold for exorbitant sums, usually to overseas buyers.

The houses in the north were often shitters. Weather battered weatherboards that were now grey and split. Sagging eves, broken and boarded windows, long rusted corrugated iron roofs, nails popped half out. The sad story of life on the west coast of Northland – a neglected and isolated part of NZ. Truth be told, the locals liked being left alone – many of them would rather be left to their own devices. It wasn't exactly lawless up there but they had their own set of laws – much like East Cape. A last Eldorado.

The dwelling that got my attention was the one made with shipping containers on two sides and wrecked cars stacked on top of each other on the other two sides. This was topped by a framework of timber and tarps. Industrious and recycling at it's finest.

The driving was like nowhere else. If Kiwis were the worst drivers in the world, then Northland drivers were the worst of the worst. Flat out and often driving death-traps. Cars that would be declared dead in many areas were kept alive in the north and put to work. Donut spare wheels were de rigeur: to be used as a regular wheel. Go hard or go home – think Kaikohe Demolition in full colour reality.

I swerved wildly as a blue ute towing a boat nearly took me out. It missed by inches. I felt like my right leg had been shaved.

I regained control and went to give a one-fingered salute and yell obscenities but the ute had gone. It was low flying. *Dirty bastard.* I was a fully paid up member of the school of 'What goes around comes around'. That prick would get his comeuppance. I would have a lot of time to contemplate Kiwi drivers over the next few weeks.

I had plenty of fire in my genes, being a Kiwi of Scottish and Irish heritage. It took some kilometres for my temper to cool after that encounter. But I didn't want it to spoil my day. *Breathe, breathe.*

'You need a firearm, son,' said Homer.

I couldn't disagree.

The Waipoua Forest began as I crested the last part of the climb. One of NZ's great forests. The home of Tane Mahuta – Lord of the forest. The giant kauri tree. Tane Mahuta held his father, Ranginui (the sky), apart from his mother, Papatuanuku (the earth). He was the go between; a lot of weight for a lone kauri to bear.

'What's all that buzzing?' asked Homer.

'It's my tinnitus,' I replied.

'No, not that noise.'

'Must be the cicadas.'

'Who's sick?'

'You.'

'Hey, am I? Wait a minute. No I'm not.'

Then a glorious downhill. Apexes, wide lines, speed. I tucked in and enjoyed the ride. At the bottom was the turnoff to the Waipoua Forest

Café. A café closed sign was screwed to a tree; there was a theme developing here.

I consulted the guide for directions – there were no other riders in sight and I needed guidance. I chose the next turn on the left to pursue. This led down to a very sweet bridge and a sign saying the road was closed.

Hmmn, I considered. *Closed, but to who? Or whom?* There were probably roads on this tour closed to many but the chosen few. The TA'ers. Or, perhaps I should head back to the main road and have a think.

Back at the intersection a TA'er flew past and waved.

'Okay, wrong turn,' I confessed.

'You think,' said Homer, needlessly

'Like you've never made one.'

'Can't recall one,' replied Homer.

'What about the time you pushed the big red button at the nuclear plant?'

'A tiny mistake. One tiny mistake.'

I could see the rider ahead turn down a road to the left. A gravel road – the first gravel of the tour.

Thank the lord. Gravel.

The gravel was splendid with little in the way of corrugation. It was mostly sweeping lines of loose stone. Sand, tiny stones right through to 20mm rocks. Gap 20 I guessed. It was kind of like surfing. Looking out at the swell and divining where the break was best. Which line of gravel to carve.

The trick with the gravel was to ride the high line if possible. The dry hard line where the stones had been swept away.

My little slice of highway heaven.

Donnellys Crossing featured a pop-up TA oasis. A coffee caravan outside an old barn converted temporarily into a cafe – tables and chairs outside.

Scones, muffins, cakes, pasta, salad – incredible. Chilli in a bowl – irresistible.

Half a dozen fellow cyclists sat around with happy faces. This was what we'd imagined the tour would consist of. Friendly accommodating cafes.

Joe, a rider who had departed from Opononi that morning, was standing in the very middle of the road looking intently into his phone. That exact point on the road was where the signal was to be found.

'There's a new Covid outbreak,' called Joe. 'Papatoetoe. There's going to be an announcement by Ashley this afternoon.'

That took a little of the wind out of our sails. Although strangely it also introduced a hint of excitement into the good ship Lollipop.

The Covid-19 virus was running rampant throughout the world but NZ was at this point isolated from its terror. However, there had been a nationwide lockdown earlier which had derailed the previous year's TA adventure leaving many short of the finishing line.

An outbreak of the virus had threatened the start of this TA but through the good work of the health department, and the use of spells and incantations, it had been shut down. Now it had reared its ugly head again. And it was ugly.

'They could lock down Auckland,' called Joe, verbalising all our fears.

I immediately went into creative combat mode. I would get one of my kids to grab the ute and the trailer and come on a rescue mission. Swoop in, sweep us up and deposit us south of the Bombays.

With difficulty I snapped my attention back to the present setting.

'I guess we just keep on going to Dargaville,' said Simon soberly. 'Then we can decide what to do.'

Right, I nodded. Cool heads.

'Dulp,' murmured Homer.

It turned out that Simon had sold a house to Ashley Bloomfield – why that had any relevance to our situation, no one could say. But it seemed terribly important right there, right then. Like we had a portal into Ashley's world: one that could set us free if it really hit the fan.

I looked around at the small group. We were in this together – they weren't the competition. They were fellow riders battling the elements, the conditions. Battling the virus. This was a time for consolidation.

Speaking of which, I went off to find the little boy's room to get rid of some consolidation. Also, to apply more butt cream. As I exited the WC, I found Simon surreptitiously doing the same.

Aha, I considered. *Even the fittest riders are getting sore butts.*

Sore butt or no, Simon was one of those riders that never seemed to tire. He would ride up the hills chatting away, usually chatting to himself as the rest of the crew were too buggered to respond. Many were chugging up in survival mode – he seemed to be powering up – recharging. *How was that possible?*

Dargaville was not far away when from out of the sun, three kids on bikes descended on me and my fellow TA'ers. *Like highway robbers.* Young ones, but still.

They were actually a trio of delightful siblings, also known as Trail Angels. People who went out of their way to supply food or drink for TA riders. The kids were being home schooled – you could tell by their sparkling eyes and radiant intelligence. They were using an app on their phones to follow the trackers the TA'ers had on-board. When their tracking apps showed a TA'er closing, they would race down the road and intercept them. *Then lure them back to their nest and tie them in silk, to be devoured at their leisure. Ha.*

The travellers were offered watermelon, water and lollies, for free – delightful.

Dargaville was just over the hill. Dargaville was a town of nearly 5,000 people.

It played small cousin to Whangārei, the city in the east. Some people in Whangārei would say unkind things about Dargaville. That it was full of hillbillies and rednecks. That it was only known for being the kumara capital. That everyone in Dargaville was related; people kept it within the family.

Mark Williams, lead singer for Dragon, inducted into the ROCKONZ Hall of Fame, came from Dargaville. Tony Quinn, the owner of racetracks, Hampton Downs, Highlands Motorsports Park and Taupō Motorsports Park, built his pet food empire from humble beginnings in Dargaville.

Still, it could be hard to change the minds of big cousins.

Dargaville to Poutu Point

44km seal, 25km gravel.

The Covid-19 outbreak had been contained. The TA could continue as planned – a huge relief to the riders.

I hadn't slept well. The previous day's ride had left me wired and unable to relax. This phenomenon wasn't uncommon and was shared by many. Riders lying on their beds, bodies exhausted but their brains swirling. An early tour experience where the brain was over stimulated after a 12-hour day and didn't know how to turn off. Some complained of headaches – dehydration was a likely culprit.

I noticed that my legs had turned to wood: they were heavy and felt like dead weight. 'This won't do at all,' I moaned. I lifted a leg and let it fall limp, weak and white. *Legs, I need you to help me. At least up the hills.* I knew this was a by-product of not being fit – however, at some point the legs would need to contribute. Especially with the mountains ahead. The first week was always going to be hard as the body got into shape.

I packed smartly then pulled a heavy can of baked beans from a pannier – my last can, thank goodness. However, the leftover Pad Tahi from last night went right into the bag, just as much dead weight. I made sure to keep the container upright so the juices wouldn't flow into his luggage.

The baked beans went down surprisingly well for breakfast. Two cups of tea and I was on my way. Most of the other riders had already left the campground. I was unperturbed as I tried to become the new me, the chilled me, the unhurried me.

I rode to the nearest hardware store for cable ties to refasten the sender unit-cum-speedo-clock-thingy. It had come loose from the front forks and I had no way of reading how slow I was going.

Dargaville was surprisingly busy. People looked sideways at me. Small-town suspicion was in the air but I dispelled this with a cheery 'Hi'. They would then break into a big grin. This made the encounters friendly and gave locals a chance to show off the teeth they owned.

The hardware store was a step back in time. A bell on the door announced arrivals. Brooms and mops in the first row, tools in the second, a wide variety of hammers. It was like visiting Arkwrights (Open all Hours) with Ronnie Barker in charge.

The goods had handwritten price tags. Photos of the founder and his staff adorned a wall. I found the cable ties and took them to the lady at the till. It was an electronic till but she did write my receipt in longhand.

Ah, I thought, *proper.*

Dargaville was prospering with the recent boom in property prices throughout NZ. Many were selling up in Auckland and looking for lifestyles in the provinces. Sell the Auckland house for an outrageous sum, buy a substantial house in Dargaville, perhaps with a big section, buy a boat and invest the rest.

The road to Poutu Point began with a long sealed straight. The occasional logging truck roared past. Much to the disgust of Homer, I got into walking mode early. It wasn't really my fault: my legs had turned to wood. The hills were short and sharp. At 44km's the road turned to gravel and it was there that the fun began.

I had been doggedly refusing to lower the tyre pressures. I had 60 lbs in the front and a little more in the back. Forty was probably the maximum recommended but I had my own theories on this – the higher the pressure the easier the wheels rolled. The downside was that the ride was a little harsh. Like riding on an old bed frame with steel casters. Not ideal with my sore butt, but.

The Poutu gravel was about as bad as you could get for a bicycle, even a mountain bike with fat knobby tyres. A hard base with marble-sized rocks. The lack of smaller stones and sand made it feel like the wheels were ricocheting off the rocks. I gritted my teeth and hung on grimly as the bike skittered about.

'Will not lower the pressure, will not lower the pressure,' I grimaced, sounding more like Homer than me.

This didn't matter on the uphills as I was walking most of them anyway. The downhills became very exciting. I stood up on the pedals to minimise the jarring and allow the bike to find its own track. The back wheel would bounce from side to side, the front skated loosely across the stones trying to find purchase. Unnerving but exciting.

The trip on the gravel was uneventful aside from falling off three times. They were slow near stationary falls. I considered them to be collateral damage with the need to maintain high tyre pressures. I embraced falling – it was one of the few things I was good at.

The logging trucks would pass leaving just enough room so that I didn't shit myself. The drivers were unfailingly courteous. However, logging truck plus gravel road equalled a shock wave of blinding, choking dust. The dust would sweep forward like fallout from a nuclear blast. I had my neck buff pulled over my face to keep the worst of it out.

The only answer was to stop completely and wait a few minutes for the dust to clear – then proceed. It was tough going and the condition of the gravel was the most difficult I would encounter on the tour.

Poutu Point was a village made up of Kiwiana baches. It looked incredibly cute and tidy after the hell of the logging road. *Who would have thought this slice of heaven was at the end of that nasty road?*

The mouth of the Kaipara Harbour was right there. Just off Poutu Point. *Probably why it was called a point.* The sea was shimmering and oily slick like mackerel skin under a hot sky.

The Kaipara Harbour laid claim to being one of the biggest harbours in the world. It was 400 square kilometres in area at low tide and more than 900 at high tide. There were some mudflats to be had in the Kaipara. It was no co-incidence the first part of its name was kai – it was a seafood basket.

TA cyclists were lazing about on the lawn next to the Marine Hall. It was a stunning day. Cold fizzy drinks and ice-creams were on sale and in hot demand at the little store.

I dismounted wearily at the bottom of the lawn. A square shouldered woman, bearing a military posture was issuing orders in a deep bass voice. She was endeavouring to instruct the TA hoi polloi on the correct manner in which to assemble for the impending ferry. Even from distance I could see that she was the boss – but she had her work cut out. The cyclists were scattered about like spent cockle shells. I pushed my bike up the lawn and joined the gathering. The dominant woman was standing on a small deck beside the hall: it was higher than the lawn; she towered over us.

(I could picture her in a grey tunic: 'You may only have your name, rank and serial number, but let me assure you, vee have vays to make you talk.')

(Actually she was very sweet and said: 'You vill all drown, die and sink to za bottom of zee ocean.')

No really, she was kind and compassionate.

The ferry was due later in the afternoon so most of the riders busied themselves with eating – a common practice on the tour. I carefully removed the leftover Pad Thai from my pannier. It hadn't spilt despite the rough road. It was slightly warm from the day's sun. I enjoyed the covetous looks from fellow riders. *Little did they know.*

The ferry duly arrived at the assigned time and TA'ers rushed about removing the bags from their bikes. The ferry was a brightly painted grand old wooden vessel. Of stubby appearance, it looked robust enough to stand up to whatever weather the Gods could throw at it.

There was no landing dock, so the skipper nudged it up to an outcrop of soft ledge and held it there on the throttle. Thank goodness there wasn't a swell running. A human chain was formed and under the guidance of the crew, the bikes were passed along and hauled up onto the top deck. It was quite a sight. People in tight bright Lycra performing synchronised moves with bikes.

Close to 50 bikes were roped down on the top level. The Surly owners took extra care with the corralling of their deluxe cycles. They regarded exclusivity as being necessary to maintain the purity of the breed. Keep the Surlys in their own pen so they could rub frames, sniff chains and generally back up to one another.

The TA riders made it safely aboard and the ferry was reversed into the broad expanse of the harbour. The skipper came over the speakers and introduced himself as Captain Wilson – he never confirmed whether this was his first or last name. He had a dry but forthright voice that rose ambitiously at the end of each sentence: very distinctive. You could have been excused for thinking Rhys Derby had taken over the wheel – a similar cheerful monotone.

It was a family affair with the first mate being his wife – the first mated they would say in Dargaville. His daughter and son-in-law were the deck hands. The first mate also doubled as the usher, stevedore, cleaner and cook. The deck hands did nothing. The wife's specialty dish was a hot dog in a bun, with pickle. It was a winning concept; the sea made one hungry.

I found a spot on a bench near the galley – I could have a good look at the preparing of the sausage. It was pleasant. To be on the sea, in the salt air and warm sun. I was pleasantly nodding off, dreaming of Thai beaches, when I felt the bench flex; a form lowering itself beside me. I partly opened my closest eye. A bearded man's face was only inches away, staring directly at me. I moved my eye slowly up and down. The man was bedecked in a startling array of new cycling gear.

Had the man noticed that I was awake?

'Robert,' said the man, extending a hand.

'Humpff, ompff,' I replied. I straightened and reluctantly opened both eyes. 'Duncan.'

'I couldn't help noticing,' enthused Robert. 'But you have Mon Royale socks.'

'Do I?' I said, surprised.

'Yes yes, you most certainly do.'

'They were a present from my daughters.'

'Well, they certainly knew what they were buying. Did you know they go right and left?'

'Ummm,' I said. My daughters did have political persuasions. 'I guess Bianca would be right. Molly would certainly be left.'

Robert looked hard at me. 'Your socks. Your socks have a left and a right foot.'

'Oh, do they?' I said, genuinely bemused. 'How would you know?'

'Well of course the left sock has the Mons on the back of it. The right has the Royale.' Robert looked well pleased. 'Did you also know, that spelt backwards, Mons says snow. And the creators didn't even know this when they designed them. Amazing.'

My heart fell. This guy was a gear-head. A sinking feeling swept over me; *not good when you're on a boat.*

'I see you've gone for the Shimano clipless shoes. What model are those?' asked Robert.

I straightened a leg out and elevated it slightly. 'They're the black ones.'

'I tried the Giro Empire WVR 90,' said Robert, elevating his leg alongside mine. 'But, like you, I went Shimano. The SH XC5. I like them *a lot.*'

'Good,' I replied. I looked around for a distraction. There was no one close that I could point to as an offering. ('Hey lookie, that fella has shiny red shoes.') Somehow, I had to escape this boffin.

'I've gone for the Gore C5 short sleeve trail jersey. Thought long sleeve but then it is February.' Robert laughed effusively showing off a perfect set of teeth. 'And the Excocets Ground Effects bib – perfect match.'

I nodded numbly, my eyes scavenging desperately for escape. It wasn't really a diatribe; it was more an earnest sermon from an evangelical cycle nut. I needed either to run or to kill myself.

'What bike are you riding?' asked Robert.

Sweet mother of mercy, I gulped. 'Look, you must excuse me,' I cheeped, and sprung to my feet. Robert was holding his helmet in his lap, one with a tiny rear-vision mirror attached to it. He looked expectantly up at me. What marvellous piece of kit was I going to show him?

I swiftly turned on my heel and made for the stern.

The trip took all of three hours and demonstrated the size of the Kaipara Harbour. In reality it could probably have been done in just 30 minutes, but Captain Wilson had the habit of killing the engine when he wished to address the passengers. And this was often. The incoming tide was rapid. It was such a powerful force that in 2008 Crest Energy received resource consent to put 200 underwater turbines into its flow.

When the skipper cut the throttle the rushing tide made the ferry bob alarmingly and it would sweep backwards at a great rate of knots. The skipper didn't sound or seem concerned by this, neither did his wife or the feckless crew.

Skipper Wilson was most informative on the amount of sand dredged from the harbour, the return of fairy terns to the sandbanks and disturbingly, the number of ships that had been wrecked at the mouth of the harbour – the number varied from 40 to more than 100 depending on who you talked to.

After a five-minute spiel on a given subject, Skipper Wilson would then throw the boat into gear and off it would valiantly chug. If it was lucky, it would make it back to the spot it had previously been before Skip would once again hit the stop button for another sermon on the sea. I suspected that Kapitan Wilson might be addicted to the Discovery channel or David Attenborough.

He demonstrated that not only was he a man with knowledge, but his sense of humour was still in good shape: 'By the way, if you need lifejackets, they are in hatches on the top deck, under the bikes,' he chortled. 'Saving your bikes will be the least of your worries. You'll have to throw them overboard to get to the life vests.'

My stomach began sending mixed messages about halfway into the voyage. I didn't speak Thai and so didn't fully understand at first. What I did understand was that I was on a slow boat with a landing still some distance away and a Pad Thai evacuation was going to be necessary. The head (the toilet) was a mission and I spent as long trying to get into the cubby as on it. At that stage it was only wind – in me. I was impressed and surprised at how much wind I had stored – its volume and especially the force of its release. Fortunately, the ferry's engine drowned out all sound.

The harbour thinned to a narrow estuary on the approach to Parakai, the drop-off point. Mangroves stretched in all directions. The bird life was prolific.

The bikes were unloaded, again using the human chain method. The first mate was well in control and the operation went smoothly. The deckhands were nowhere to be seen. Skipper Wilson bade everyone bon voyage over the intercom. My shipmates and I never did get to see him. He never came out from the wheelhouse.

It was sunset so riders set up their bikes for night riding. Most had accommodation booked nearby. A bunch of us decided it was such a nice evening that riding into Auckland City was the go. The temperature was still warm enough that only one layer was needed. There was the added advantage that traffic would be light at that time of the night.

Helensville to Auckland City

32km sealed roads, 16km sealed cycleway

It was a beautiful night for a ride. A full moon, no wind and very few cars. When you considered that it would be gridlock come the morning, the decision to ride through the night was a good one and of course there was the entertainment. I provided the entertainment; not willingly.

Every 30 minutes or so, I would screech to a halt and tear off into the nearby bush. An Asian take on Montezuma's revenge.

'Cheeseburger and fries pal,' lectured Homer, as I pulled myself back onto the bike. 'Stick to burger and fries. God's food.'

It was basically just hot air that I was expelling. Many wouldn't have been surprised by this, but it sure was an exorbitant amount of methane even by a cow's standard. A small hole was burned in the ozone that night.

The balmy night held with us as we pedalled the Old North Rd. *What's with the Old? Old North Rd, Old Coach Road – must be one of those in every province. Old Ghost Rd.* I had enough on my plate without those contemplations.

The 16km cycleway into Auckland City began near Kumeū. A wide, well-lit piece of pavement that was well patronised during the day. At that time of night, it was empty and the group only passed one cyclist. Bed at 2am.

Auckland

Pad Thai rest day

I took it easy and slowly worked my way into the day. I stayed with the Thai theme and ended up on my front receiving a Thai massage. The masseuse spent most of the hour working on my calves. I practised holding my breath and not screaming.

I basically did nothing during the day but lounge about – and shop. I was staying at my sister's in Onehunga, which was close to Rouleur Cycles. I didn't know that this was one of NZ's premier cycle shops. It wasn't far from the Thai massage studio. I stumbled through the door, my calves completely useless. I didn't know whether they hurt more before or after the Thai pummelling.

I needed two drink bottle cages, as I was ditching my frame bag. One cage would hold the lighter fuel for the stove, the other would hold a bottle of electrolyte. It was a shame to get rid of my frame bag but it had flunked. I had built it and while the bag itself was fine, the double-sided Velcro had failed. The frame bag had made my bike look a little like speedway legend, Ivan Mauger's speedway bike – that would be missed.

The chap at the counter was appalled that I had chosen two different styles of bottle cage. I was horrified at the price of everything. The plastic bottles were the same price as the bottle cages; carrying water could be an expensive exercise.

'You've got two different cages mate,' said the staffer holding them up. 'Are they going on the same bike?'

'Yes,' I replied.

'Orr, you can't do that. It'll look like dog's balls.'

'I would take that as a compliment. If I was a dog,' I said.

The staffer blinked at me, not computing.

'They do different jobs,' I explained. 'One of the bottles holds electrolyte, the other holds meths.' I leaned closer to the staffer and knowingly touched the side of my nose. 'You know, a small slug in the arvo to keep your senses on point.' I couldn't help myself.

The staffer blinked again. Was this man attempting humour on him?

He came out from behind the counter. He was clearly a cyclist: his legs were long, well defined and hairless.

I could do with a pair of those, I thought.

The staffer tried to sell hydration tablets to me. He tried to sell gels and pastes to offset any cramp. I wasn't buying. The prices were outrageous. These products were wasted on me – I was no athlete.

I was clearly in the wrong store. I should never have gone into one of the most techy bicycle stores in the country. I looked around and wondered whether there was a Warehouse nearby.

The staffer had one last go at selling to me. He enquired as to what bike I was using for the TA. When I said it was a Giant XTC 29er that I'd got for $800 second-hand, the staffer just stared at me blankly; for a long time.

Could this fella be some kind of cyborg?

The staffer, the cyborg, appeared to come up with a blank on my breed of bike. A bike for under $1000 didn't exist in any category that he knew – *this was Rouleur Cycles.* He had definitely come up with a blank on me – I wasn't your typical cyclist.

The staffer ushered me to a stand in the middle of the store. There, was a Cannondale Topstone Carbon – possibly the best gravel bike ever made. It would be perfect for the Tour Aotearoa. It would be fast. What's more, you could get extras for it.

It was $14,000; without the extras.

I also shopped at the Onehunga Mall and bought two new shirts. Ones that wouldn't chafe my nipples.

Auckland to Miranda Hot Springs

103km sealed roads, 4km gravel

I felt better after a day's rest. Pad Thai would be off the menu for the rest of the tour but it was now time to get back on the bike.

Like most big cities Auckland was a place where getting out of was more difficult than getting in. I was still using the TA official guide to navigate, which was mostly fine. However, it was a couple of years out of date and Auckland's road network was a constantly changing beast – the proliferation of road cones didn't help. In fact, the country was being held hostage by the bloody coners.

Conspiracy theorists were saying that the cones were multiplying in response to the rollout of 5G. Proline Plastics, the leading manufacturer of road cones was making 50,000 cones a year. Each one weighed five kilograms and had a life span of five years. I felt like I'd personally met each and every one of them.

Downer traffic services manager, Jon Atherton, looked after 12,000 cones and reckoned it was challenging. People deliberately opened their car doors to knock down hundreds of lines of perfectly placed cones. *Oh, the urge, the urge.* I was somehow gratified to know that others braver than me had given into it. Lord knows I had been close to the *knock em over* flashpoint many times; who hadn't. It was just so tempting, those orderly lines of orange blighting the country. Coners with careful intensity positioned them arrow straight. And the sheer number of them used on each site. However, if you were getting $1.50 per cone, per day, you too would be laying them down thick.

NZTA admitted to spending $768 millon on the road insanity and out of control. Sorry, that should read, safety and control. That figure didn't include the price of the cones.

An element of 'tomfoolery with drunken students' was being blamed for cones going missing. Who didn't have one in the back yard? But there was talk of a 'recent shift change' where small contractors were poaching the unguarded cones at night. At $31 to buy a cone you could see why they would be tempting under the new age of health and safety requirements.

I had used the rest day to load a new app on my phone for guidance – CampMate. It was a lovely day for cycling. I sat astride my bike and began scanning.

John, from Tuakau, was offering free accommodation. Mike, next door in Pokeno, was keen to do some tenting next weekend. Stuart (Stuballs) was setting up his pop-up in Miranda. The "Backstreet Boys" from Hamilton were having their annual picnic in Clevedon.

I rubbed my eyes in confusion. Was I looking at this correctly? This wasn't what I expected.

'I think the correct term at this stage is, *Dulp*!' called Homer, breaking in on my investigation. 'You did say you were looking for adventure.'

'What do you mean?' I asked.

'I think you may be heading up the wrong alley, so to speak,' speculated Homer.

I hit Google to try to find out what was going on.

'Dulp. You are right. Crikey, little buddy. That could have become awkward.' I looked skywards and slowly shook my head. I could still amaze myself. 'If you add e-r, you get Campermate. Campmate: that would be a camp, as in gay, site.'

I did some quick deleting and reloading.

CamperMate – although it was really for those with motorhomes, I figured it could be perfect for cycle tourists too. Plus, it did cover all of the far reaches of NZ. I felt sure it would be useful and keep my bacon intact.

My legs were changing. They weren't ready for the Tour de France yet but the blood now seemed to be going through them rather than stopping at them. The quads were sore and the calves were fresh to the touch, but ready to become part of the team – to join the tour.

Mangere Bridge had a cycleway clip-on sheltered under its wing. I had ridden this before. I stopped at its entrance and a bunch of women cyclists surged past and onto the bridge path. It was Saturday and Aucklanders were out to play. The old Mangere Bridge was to the right. Cars with boats behind were in an orderly queue waiting to use the boat ramp. Unload the boat and file back along the bridge to the carpark. A cracker day to be on the water. No breeze at that stage and a bright sky.

There was one other chap on a bike waiting patiently as the women filed onto the bridge lane. I hadn't noticed him before which was surprising as the man was staggeringly drunk – no easy feat when on a bicycle, especially at eight in the morning. The drunk and I poised ready to follow the women. The drunk launched before me but after one stroke of his pedal his foot slipped and he toppled to the side.

One down, I sniggered and shot past him. The cycle route, Kiwi Esplanade, went around the suburb called Mangere Bridge and it was well used. The new motorway bridge with the clip-on cycleway was called Mangere Bridge. The old bridge, which was now mostly for fishing access, was called Mangere Bridge. *What could possibly go wrong?* Warning signals should have been clanging in my brain.

I got myself lost almost immediately. Emerging from the covered bridge clip-on I found the female peloton had given me the slip: too quick. I wound in and out of the local streets, the guide in one hand, my eyes squinting with effort trying to read the street names. No surprise that this system of navigation wasn't working. Still, I was not one to give up.

With the use of the guide and by following other random cyclists, I managed to get myself onto Kiwi Esplanade and heading in the right direction.

The trail led past what had affectionately been known for years as the 'Puhinui Poo Ponds'. It was now called the Mangere Lagoon. (The pen is mightier than the sword – or shovel.) But there was no hiding the sweet smell of sewage. The surrounding land had been turned into cycle and walking trails, a pony club and a park. A haven.

Papatoetoe was the suburb where the latest Covid-19 outbreak was blooming. It was also where a massive amount of road work was underway. Coners had been enthusiastically about their work. I weaved in and out of large orange cones. The workmen had been kind enough to keep the cycleway open by using the cones.

It took two hours to negotiate my way from the Auckland metropolis into the countryside. I stopped at a roadside store at Alfriston to catch my breath and to buy blueberries – antioxidants. It had been a shit of a ride. Trying to get out of Auckland was like trying to crawl out of a puddle of sago.

The upside was that, using my new app, I could locate every campervan dumpsite in South Auckland. What a waste of time. I clicked on the CamperMate app and pushed delete; yet another jettisoned app.

The road to the east coast was popular, especially with boaties. It had no shoulder and I battled valiantly to stay on its edge while boat trailers swished past. To be fair, most of the drivers were doing their best to give me room, there just wasn't much. It was exhausting, living on the edge of the road like that.

I put in my earbuds and tuned into a podcast. One featuring NZ motocross legend, Ben Townley. Townley was one of those Kiwis that threw some clothes in a suitcase, borrowed a few bucks from Mum, and set off to have a crack at racing bikes on the other side of the world. He was good and ended up competing in the motocross world championships – culminating in him winning the 2004 MX2 world championship. Ben then went to the USA and raced for eight years in the American motocross championship.

'Now there's a fella who's lived on the edge,' I said.

'Yep,' agreed Homer. 'Did you know that boy was teammate in the states with Ricky Carmichael? The GOAT. Greatest of all time.'

I squinted at Homer. 'Didn't know you were into motocross pal.'

'There's a lot of things you don't know about me. Pal.'

'True that.'

'I may be just a doll screwed down to these bars to you. But I've been around. Mate.'

'Come on Homes, I know you are special.' I took a hand off the bars and put it over his mouth. 'Special needs,' I muffled.

'I heard that,' shouted Homer. Then he chortled. 'Probably why we are together on this ridiculous journey. We both have special needs.'

It was nice for me to take my mind away from the impending thoughts of being hit from behind by a car.

One bonus about being in the thick of the traffic was that there were cafes open. A veritable feast of them. An omelette and a vanilla milkshake were no problem – even multiple milkshake stops were possible. Also a chance to top up, bottom up, my butt cream applications.

The coastal road ran beside the Firth of Thames, a gem of a road. Baches were tucked neatly into bends in the road. It was winding with gentle rises and falls – perfect cycling geography and the momentum could be maintained.

There was a row of uniform white buildings I could just make out on a distant peninsula. On drawing closer I realised they were in fact motorhomes – nose to tail and gleaming brightly in the sunshine. A freedom camping site right on the water; NZ was blessed with these sites.

Miranda Hot Springs was the destination for the night. Soothe the aching legs in the healing waters. The campground was chocka but the chap in the office found room for my wee pup tent. $28 for the night. I didn't spot any other TA'ers at the campground. My day off in Auckland meant that those in my group were now a day's ride ahead.

First stop was a dip in the natural hot pool in the campground. Being a weekend it was busy with family groups.

I hadn't shaved since beginning the tour. The unshaven look was trendy but I was no stud. I also had odd tan lines from my bike apparel: mid-shin to just above the knee were tan and the rest of my legs were Anglo-Saxon white. I wore my bike chamois shorts in the pool to give them a rinse. (The overall look could be described as "cycle gimp"). Parents gently corralled their children away to other reaches of the pool.

Whatever, I thought and gently corralled a fart, allowing it to mushroom my shorts briefly before bursting for the surface. A faint smell of Pad Thai wafted by.

Dinner was beef burger and chips. Again. To be honest there weren't many choices. There was a takeaway caravan set up by the office in the campground and that was the only source of cooked food.

'I see you're back on the good stuff pal,' said Homer. 'Uncle Sam's finest.'

I was in bed by dark, earplugs in and soon asleep.

9.50pm and my phone roared to life with a tsunami warning. I, sprang upright, thrashing wildly and groping for the surface. *Must get to the air … the air.* I quickly realised I was in a tent. *But what was that racket?*

Phones were going off all over the campground. It was a Covid cacophony. Alert, alert! Auckland had gone into a level 3 lockdown due to the outbreak in Papatoetoe. A border was being put in place at 6am the following morning from the Bombay Hills to Ōrere Point, just north of Miranda Hot Springs.

I was safely south of this but for those to the north it would become a sprint to get across the border in time. Ha, Auckland became our Trump Mexico wall.

Miranda Hot Springs to Te Aroha

2km sealed road, 80km gravel

A campground mens' toilet block can be a hideous but curious start to a day. I was in there early and was joined by a couple of other early starters: *rhymes with....* The sounds could have been mistaken as coming from a zoo – the hyenas and warthogs coming awake. Little grunts followed by sighs. Then coughs, belches, groans and the stamping of feet. I wasn't sure about the stamping of feet but I did recognise the other noises: the morning ritual of men unblocking themselves.

I set sail and got the legs turning under a promising sunrise. There was a series of stop banks running towards Thames. The trail ran atop them. The birdlife was splendid in the marshes bordering the banks – home to 40,000 birds, most of them waders. The mudflats, shell banks, grass flats, saltmarsh and mangrove formed an important habitat for the shorebirds. Many of them were migratory: bar-tailed godwits and knots. The migrating birds would arrive in spring from places as far away as Siberia and Alaska. In autumn they would fly north while the natives moved in: pied oystercatchers and wrybills.

The stop banks gave a great view down the Firth of Thames. The track was flat, enjoyable and cruisy riding.

I wasn't sure what navigation system to use this day, what with the failure of CamperMate. The TA guidebook made it look pretty straightforward as the Hauraki Rail Trail tracked down the middle of the North Island. You just had to stay on it. That couldn't be hard.

As I came to the Piako River, Pipiroa, a delightful older chap had his van parked and he was waiting. He informed me that he was keeping a log of numbers coming through. He also pointed which way to go. This was unnecessary as it was even obvious to me as there was only one lane across the bridge. But it was a nice thing to do.

Soon after however, there was a T junction in the path. I looked about and spotted a rider, ahead a few hundred metres. I too quickly reverted to my earlier method of following anyone on a bike. *You couldn't really get lost that way as that person was heading somewhere, weren't they?*

The rider turned out to be a man wearing long shorts and a chequered shirt. As I caught up to him the man suddenly stopped. I pulled up beside him. We both looked ahead to what appeared to be the end of the trail – at least a serious thinning of it.

'Do you know where this heads?' the man enquired.

'No, I thought you did,' I said, grimacing slightly. So much for my theory.

'No, I'm not from around here,' enthused the stranger. 'Oh well.' And he cheerfully mounted up and turned back in the direction we'd just come from.

'For feck's sake,' I groaned.

Back to the T junction and take the only other turn. It has taken me most of my life to realise that I usually made the wrong decision. If it was a 50/50 call I always guessed wrong. Take an example: picking up a pair of undies in the dark and putting them on. Always back to front. Of course I could guess wrong, but not take the guess and go the other way. But that would be double jeopardy and then you wouldn't know if you were Arthur or Martha. It was best to just resign oneself to being wrong.

The NZ cricket team under Kane Williamson had lost all five coin tosses on its recent trip to India, so I wasn't the only one struggling with luck. And the working theory in India was that if you lost the toss you lost the test. Former captain Brendon McCullum had a record of 10 tosses won and 16 lost in test cricket.

Somehow I negotiated my way across the busy road leading to Thames and got onto the cycle path on the other side.

The Hauraki Rail Trail. No fighting traffic today for me, no sir. A 200km trail that cost a fortune to build. Studies found that the mean spend per cyclist who used the trail was about $100. Extrapolated out it meant that the Hauraki Trail generated a spend of two to three million dollars per year. It was mostly used by Aucklanders. The trail ran predominantly through the flat farmland of the Hauraki Plains. Farmers had to be persuaded that it was a good thing in allowing their farms to be used as a corridor for cycling. Fences were built on both sides of the trail. Gates installed where farmers needed to move cows. Ground prepared, built up and flattened. Many truckloads of metal spread on the trail. Swing bridges built over gullies and streams. The end result was a wide, flat pathway that was so monotonous it was hard to believe anyone would ride it.

It was no 90 Mile Beach but to my butt it felt similar. The same gear the same cadence, the same rub-dee-rub of the sit bones.

It beats riding the main road I accepted. But it was in the same league as taking six of the best being preferable to doing detention.

Paeroa was a welcome sight and a chance to get off the trail.

'Hey Homer, wake up,' I called. 'Last time I rode a bike through Paeroa I was doing over 200 klicks down the main street and I didn't get arrested. It was The Battle of the Streets races.'

'Well thank the lord I didn't know you then,' replied Homer. 'God knows what you could have put me through.'

The Battle of the Streets motorcycle races had been a regular feature on the NZ racing calendar when I was a bona fide motorbike racer. Unfortunately, due to a host of factors, the event was no longer – and unlikely to return. I had raced a Suzuki GSXR1100 in the Post Classic class. The 'posties' class consisted of bikes built before 1990 and most of them were heavy, unwieldy lumps of metal. To make them fast wasn't so hard: with access to race pistons, camshafts, carbs and a bit of trick internal work. To make them handle was a different matter – you certainly felt your oats trying to ride one.

The Paeroa track was short but it was the fastest one of NZ's street circuits. Street circuits, by their nature, were filled with manmade obstacles: manhole covers, zebra crossings, even railway crossings. Then there were the potholes, crests and kerbs. Paeroa was unique in that the back straight had two roads that joined it – there were large humps in the road where they joined. These provided 'jumps' for the riders and, depending on how brave they were, how much air they got. It was a popular place for spectators.

The front straight had a slight left kink in it – the average motorist wouldn't notice it at 50kph. However, at around 200kph it was significant. It became a one-line corner: no room for two bikes. Tucked down behind the screen, I had the throttle pinned – this was no place for sissies – it was a place to make time. Braking markers were set on the left-hand side of the road. Just before the 100-metre sign, I would slide my bum to the right for the turn, nip the brake lever in and then squeeze it hard while simultaneously going down three gears. Strangely, the butt was a marvellous gauge for dictating how hard one could brake, along with the feet and the hands. The back wheel would skip and lift on the asphalt, even pulling the bike from side to side. The trick was to get it under control and find that magic word, stability. Time could be made on the brakes. Then knee out and throw it on its side, look through the corner and give it enough gas to hold the line. The corner rose sharply, turned right and plunged downhill. I hugged the kerb all the way round it, kneepad grinding the road. (Nick Cole would run his knee slider along the top of the kerbing.) I liked to stay far right, still in second gear and go briefly up to full throttle. Then hard on the front brake again and fight the bastard for control. There was a big depression just before the left turn. The bike hit the bottom of its suspension with a crunch, the fairing leaving a fibreglass smear. Then hard left, quickly followed by a hard right – a favourite overtaking place of mine: riders didn't expect you to try it on there.

I used the middle of the road down the back straight – avoided the high points of the jumps: the thought of getting it wrong on the jumps terrified me (the crowd was perched right to the edge of the footpath – only some deer fencing separating it). Throttle pinned, tucked down, bum raised slightly off the seat and standing lightly on the pegs over the jumps – shifting gears. There was a slight right before the last corner. At the apex was a manhole cover. There was just enough room to go inside it – most chose the outside route. I rode right over it; it was just something I did. The last corner brought the bike nearly to a stop. It was so tight it was more a motocross than road racing corner. Stop and go – back on the gas and climb up the bike to put weight on the front to keep it from wheelieing too much – just enough for some crowd pleasure but not enough to lose time.

'Ah, those were the days,' I said, a wistful look on his face. 'The crazy thing is that this is Highway One. The nation's main road down the country. And we got to use it as a racetrack. Yep, never felt more alive than racing on the street.' Indeed, street racing was my favourite form of the sport. The danger factor was much higher than racing on a prepared motor racing circuit.

'Adrenalin, what a drug,' I smiled. 'But for now, an omelette and a vanilla milkshake will have to do. Then we must up and away, my good friend.'

'Yep, up and away,' agreed Homer. There was a pause. 'Lost you for a moment there, buddy.'

'Yes you did,' I answered. 'Yes you did. Takes a moment to come back from those places.'

The TA guide directed the rider to go over a highway bridge and squeeze through a barrier. *Odd*, I thought. *Perhaps that direction has been outdated.* It was much easier to just follow the majority of people on bikes who were heading west, down a well-defined trail.

The trail proved popular with family groups out enjoying the cycling. Tots on three wheelers with Mum and Dad. Electric bikes were popular, even if half of those riding them could have done with the exercise of a manual bike.

Still, this was nice. The Ohinemuri River cut dramatically through the Karangahake Gorge. The rail trail followed it and its sweeps and curves. Arches of tree branches overhead dappled the sun. It was pleasantly warm.

The piece de resistance of this section of trail was the 1,100-metre-long railway tunnel. The sign said a light should be used on your bike but I could see the far end, the exit of the tunnel. It also had some limited lighting so I could stay onboard even with the occasional wobble. The tunnel had a gradual uphill feel. *Fantastic. Now we are having some fun on the trail* – after a week of graft; the body and brain adjusting to life on the road. Finally, things were becoming fun and interesting – a great piece of track to ride.

At Waikino I stopped, unease rising in me. *I was having too good a time.* I pulled the guide from the front bag and suspiciously leafed through it. Sure enough, no mention of a Paeroa to Waihi stage: I was off track. I was on a beaten track, but not the right one. I was no Tonto and this tracking method was not working.

A couple of hours of backtracking and I got myself back on course. The seemingly endless drudgery of the Hauraki Rail Trail became my life again.

By Te Aroha I had had enough of that day's cycling. Plus, the Te Aroha campground had a hot pool. Te Aroha was quiet being a Sunday.

'This place is like a ghost town,' said Homer nervously, his big eyes bugging. 'You sure we're safe here?'

'Pretty sure, Homey. Don't know much about it – it's off the beaten track.'

'Oohh, worse,' snivelled Homer.

'Relax, mate. This isn't America.'

'I don't want to relax. And don't call me Homey.'

Te Aroha was a substantial sized town of 4000 people. Historic buildings were the main features of Te Aroha. The Te Aroha Borough Council Chamber, The Grand Tavern and the Post Office to name a few. Historic in NZ meant more than 100 years old. In Europe that would be considered just a baby – not even a toddler. Recent earthquakes had meant that old buildings in NZ were under threat of being knocked down and replaced with 'earthquake-proof' buildings. I was mortified that this was happening. I had built a cob house – it was not 100 years old, but it was built in the style of houses that were thousands of years old. There were 60,000 cob houses in County Devon alone, the youngest being 500 years old. *You can't knock down your history.*

Te Aroha was tucked beneath the steep Kaimai Ranges and probably received little sun in the winter, I reckoned, looking up at the towering hills. The gas station was open and I popped in there for a flavoured milk. A four square was also open and I bought mince and Ben's Spiced Rice for dinner – a cook up.

The Te Aroha campground was a few km's out of town; I didn't need the extra pedalling with tired legs. I also didn't need to find out there were no cabins available, I was in the mood for a proper bed.

The cabins were being used as temporary but long-term accommodation for people of no fixed abode.

I paid $25 to the camp boss and went to find an area for my tent. I sat on the ground putting the tent poles together. Bogun drifters and their red-headed, tattooed girlfriends lounged about outside the cabins. It felt like I had been transported to America and some back woods hillbilly Hicksville – *who knew these kind of places existed in NZ?*

Bang – a shot went off. Boguns with guns. I grabbed the tent tightly to my chest and scuttled behind a tree.

Pow – another shot.

I peeked around the side of the tree. The boguns and redheads were still lying about outside their cabins – some leaning against their beater cars. None of them seemed perturbed by the shooting.

How rough is this place? They're not even bothered by the sound of gunfire.

'Too rough for us,' said Homer. 'Keep your head down, pal and let's make a run for it.'

Pow-pow.

'Perhaps there's a gun club next door,' I offered. 'You can't just be firing off guns in New Zealand…. Can you?'

'That would be a negative,' replied Homer. 'Now, if we were in the good ole US of A, we wouldn't be hiding like this. We would be armed.'

'Ow,' I yowled. 'What hit me?' I reached to my head. Something hard had hit me. 'Ow.' This time I was hit in the shoulder. The projectile bounced to the ground. It was an acorn.

'Ha, it's acorns,' I laughed, my voice weak with relief. 'Falling acorns hitting the corrugated iron roofs of the cabins.'

'I knew that,' said Homer. 'I wasn't worried.'

'Yeah, right. You were just relying on me, being the bigger target – getting taken out first.'

Blimey, what a sound. Acorn season.

The acorn trees were huge and all about the campground. I did a readjustment in site choosing and put my little tent up in open ground. Away from the acorn trees. I then grabbed my towelette, a pathetic excuse for a towel – the downside of having to downsize in the packing. More like a facecloth but made of a fabric that dried quickly. A fabric that was in truth non-absorbent – it more or less just wiped the water off the body; needs must. I stripped to my shorts.

The hot pool was large and clean. Impressive. The other bonus was that no one else was using it, as in, no children were in it splashing and screaming. *Bliss – But wait. Shouldn't there be steam coming off the water?*

I edged closer and dipped a foot in. The campground had clearly advertised that it had natural hot pools.

Miffed but remaining calm, I internalised my anger and padded from the pool and quietly closed the pool gate – I didn't slam it. I made the walk across the open field, my towelette in hand, along with my dignity. Back to the tent.

That was probably light entertainment for the boguns. The day's fool who thought the pool would be hot.

Two TA'ers arrived and began setting up their camp, near the shower block. I said hello and cautioned that the hot pool was in fact cold. They were young and said they were taking their time, the ride was going to be like a honeymoon. *Whatever the hell that meant.*

The couple had hit the border checkpoint at Orere Point but had no problem getting through. One of them lived in Christchurch and the other in Wanaka. Because they lived south of Auckland, they could leave the city. Doing it by bike was a cause of consternation to the border guards, they said. But technically they had every right to go through.

'Kind of, like, if you're South Korean, you have the right to go to North Korea,' I said. 'Hey, I'm Korean. It's still Korea, isn't it?'

I smiled at the two youngsters, pleased with my comparison.

They gave one another a secret look and indicated to me that they needed to get their tent set up.

I had dinner to prepare anyway.

Mince a la rice. Basically, mince fried brown and boiled rice added, with seasoning. The seasoning was the flavour in the Uncle Ben's rice. You could choose Mexican, Chinese, Sweet and Sour. Not Korean.

A couple of the boguns joined me in the kitchen. One was a tall ginga. There were cookers and some pots. But no cutlery or crockery, which appeared to be the norm at campgrounds these days.

Fortunately, I had my Trangia pot to use as a dish and my plastic fork. It was a bright orange fork with a spoon on the other end and a serrated knife edge on one side. It was called a Spork – and it actually worked well.

The boguns were nice fellas, as were nearly all the people I met in the campgrounds of NZ. *Just because you're a bogun doesn't mean you can't be a nice one. But weren't boguns supposed to drive Holdens or Falcons? Or Zephyrs. Those were the boguns of my era*, I reflected. The modern bogun drove a shitty little Japanese car.

The ginga bogun informed me that he was the camp cleaner. He studied me for a reaction to this confession.

'The place is very tidy,' I replied. And it was – I wasn't lying. 'You have your work cut out, though, eh, as this place isn't getting any younger.'

The ginga bogun agreed and said he was looking for better work.

WW3 continued into the night as acorn trees shed their load. The boguns did what boguns do – they kept the music loud. Their laughter and talking louder. Around midnight the party finally sizzled out.

I had gone early for earplugs and a sleeping pill. However, heavy trucks started rumbling past the campground at 4am. A siren went off at 5am.

Was this another Covid warning of some sort, I wondered, groggily. I searched on my phone for Te Aroha, siren. No, it was no Covid warning. It was a time siren that was an historical feature of Te Aroha, built by Mr Bill Kean and his son, Verdon. They were from Balclutha and brought the siren north with them when they moved to Te Aroha in 1946. It was originally powered by a Chev engine.

Well, bugger me.

Te Aroha to Arapuni

63 sealed road, 13km gravel

I got myself back to the town of Te Aroha without a truck running me over; always a good start to the day. The half-light of sunrise was a dangerous time to be cycling. I had no decent headlight – my only reliable light was a small red taillight, with a flicker feature.

Once in Te Aroha I almost immediately became lost. I found where I had entered the town the day before, but that was no help. An older couple were out for a morning walk and the woman was very helpful. She pointed me in the right direction and said to look out for a 'bright white' concrete pathway. The man wore a slightly suspicious look that I was becoming familiar with.

My bike had a length of Marley drainpipe clamped to the frame – bags, flags and jandals attached in different attitudes. This was a one-off bike. It was an assortment of odds and sods with the bicycle as a platform. I was bedecked in a white and black windbreaker, camo shorts over a pair of chamois shorts, rainbow Alpinestars gloves, purple socks and black bike shoes.

I had a brief moment of self-awareness: *the campground boguns were a little out of the ordinary, but take a look at yourself, pal.*

The cycleway was indeed 'bright and white', as the woman had said. It looked to be freshly laid concrete and ran beside the highway for a long way. *It must have cost a small fortune to lay and once again, why?* Why not spend the money on building some cool trails in the Kaimai Ranges? Not on a road beside a road. For anyone who's cycled on a path beside a road, it's often a fake feeling.

Rain was falling on the top of the Kaima's. It was only light cloud over the Hauraki Plains and the weather didn't appear threatening. No wind, cool; good cycling weather. *Shame it's such a trudge but hey, beats working.* I got my cadence under control, butt fully creamed, and set sail towards Matamata.

There was a café, carefully positioned, about halfway to Matamata. That was one bonus of the Hauraki Rail Trail: there were a good number of cafes. This one was down a deep gravel driveway. I turned a little too quickly, dug the front wheel in and toppled slowly to the ground. My fourth fall. All had been on gravel and all were slow.

Falling, my forte, I conceded, as I unclipped my foot from the pedal cleat and dragged myself out from under the bike. The crucial trick is, don't put your arm out when you fall. That's a broken collarbone or arm. Keep your arm tucked in like a chicken wing and take it with the shoulder.

I was a veteran of the slow fall.

I pulled the bike upright and wheeled it to rest against a tree while I sought out what was on offer in the café. Frappes, smoothies, smushies, frittatas, vegan stacks, carrot-sugar-snap-pea and soba noodles. No milkshakes – no omelettes. The downside of the cafes on the Hauraki Rail Trail was that they were a little trendy with their menus.

I took time out to book a room at the Arapuni Backpackers, my planned destination for the night: I needed a proper bed and a catchup on some sleep.

The run to Matamata was uneventful. It was all cycle trail which made me happy. I wasn't feeling particularly energetic after the night's busyness. This was an easy navigation as there was only one path – no strain on the brain.

A TA'er was stopped near the entrance to Matamata. He was by the curb, rummaging in the front bag of his bike.

'What's the mattermatter?' I asked, pulling up beside him.

'What's that?' replied the man, head still down.

'What's the mattermatter?' I repeated; not quite as funny the second time around.

'Oh, nothing,' came a mutter. The man was unresponsive to my great wit but he did finally look up and acknowledge me. He gave me a quick up and down. 'Where are you headed?'

'To Bob's Bikes,' I said, thankful for at least being acknowledged. 'I want to get my seat looked at.'

The man briefly considered this, a grave crinkle to his brow. 'Right, I'll join you. I'm looking for a new wingman,' he said. 'I had two and now I have none. Lost them.'

'Oh, sorry to hear that. Is that what you were searching for in your bar bag?' I chuckled. *My wingman was only 70mm tall.*

The man looked hard at me.

Does this man have no sense of humour? I wondered.

'The first wingman was a doctor friend of mine.'

This could be some kind of distortion of the time continuum, I considered. *Like a two-second gap on the toll call.*

'Lost him at the Onehunga Mall.' The man peered off vacantly, as if to a distant horizon.

I sensed this man had a vagueness about him. Certainly, a distracted air. He was a tall man. He reminded me of Basil Fawlty, from *Fawlty Towers*. It probably wasn't surprising that he could lose someone; Basil was always losing things.

'Did he turn up?' I enquired, politely.

'No, no, I didn't actually lose him,' replied the man, somewhat brusquely. 'His body packed up. He couldn't go on.' He sucked a little air through his teeth, looked away again, to the hills. 'He was taking massive doses of steroids and it was all too much. He cooked himself. Had to pull out.'

'Okay,' I said, slowly, wondering about the massive doses of steroids. 'So, what happened to the other wingman?'

'His wife came and took him,' he said, a surprised note to his voice.
'What do you mean,"*took him*?"'
'When the Covid-19 alarm went off we were in the Hunua Ranges. Staying at a B and B. We had to pack the bags and ride through the night to get over the border before 6am.' The man looked pained, he sucked more air through his teeth – peered again to the horizon.

I swivelled my head and also gazed, away to the distant horizon. However, I couldn't see much aside from a couple of trees and a house. Didn't have my horizon spectacles on. *Spectacles, testicles, distant horizons* (that didn't riff).

Must concentrate and find out what this guy is about. I snapped back to the present.

'His wife drove down to Hunua and took him. She said it was ridiculous to be doing the TA at this time.' The man let out a long sigh, almost mournful. 'He was a real bonus. A little eccentric, but interesting.'

His wife had swept in like a pterodactyl and uplifted the poor chap, despite his protestations. He had been keen to continue and was having the time of his life. The Covid-19 border sprint had added even more excitement.

'So now I'm without a wingman,' said the man, swinging his gaze from the distant horizon and round to me. There was an odd light in his eyes. He smiled; for the first time. 'I'm looking for a new one. Luigi's the name. Luigi Collins.' He thrust a hand towards me.

'I'm Duncan. DC for short,' I said, shaking Luigi's hand while wondering just what being a wingman meant. *It didn't sound that successful a position.*

'I'm sorry about your wingmen,' I said, sincerely. 'Especially the second one. You can always get another wife – you can't always get another wingman.'

Luigi looked to me, a smile again breaking his face.

We cycled together to Bob's Bikes while I explained to Luigi that I wasn't great with the navigation side of things and tended to get lost, often. I figured this would put Luigi off for a while and give me some breathing room and time to discover more of the role of a wingman.

I felt like my butt was often sliding forward, slipping off the front of the saddle. I explained this to the mechanic. There was constant weight on my wrists: my arms would tingle, then go numb, if I maintained one position for too long. I had to keep shifting back.

I was looking to Bob's Bikes for another spacer to lift the handlebar stem, to take some weight off my arms.

The mechanic took one look at my bike and commented that he wouldn't ride a bike like that. That seemed a little rude to me. So, it wasn't to everyone's tastes, but my bike was certainly original. One of a kind. With relief, I realised the mechanic was talking about the seat. The saddle was fine but it was pitched on an angle too far forward. That was putting too much weight on the arms. He also pointed out that there wasn't room on the stem for another spacer. But, by lifting the nose of the seat, the problem could be solved – and it cost nothing. The mechanic was quite taken with my drainpipe drinking setup so in the end it was a win-win for me.

A couple of other fellas, John and Mike, were also at Bob's. Fellow TA riders. That made a group of four of us: plenty of wingman candidates.

'I've lost a couple of wingmen,' said Luigi, to John and Mike. 'But I think I've found a new one.' He grinned and looked to me.

I grinned weakly back – what are you going to do? I had somehow passed a recruitment test without actually volunteering or going through an employment process.

'He's not great on the navigation, gets lost easily, but no matter,' smiled Luigi. 'Those things can be fixed.'

I felt a little like the last cattle beast at an auction. The one that no one really wanted but was eventually sold. I looked to the other two fellas. Surely they were better candidates.

John was a strong looking man, into his 70s, and had road cyclist's legs. Mike was portly and didn't look like a cyclist. They weren't a team but just happened to be in Bob's shopping at the same time. Four individual men who some would say were in their prime. *Some would say a lot of things.*

It was kind of nice to be cycling with a crew again. I challenged Mike to a freewheeling contest. At the top of a hill, no pedalling, and let the bike freewheel down: find out who was faster.

I had competed in a few of these since the start of the TA. At first it had just happened because there was a big group of riders often cresting the hill together. I would easily slip by the others and always made the bottom of the hill first. This then became a test.

Mike was some ways heavier, bigger boned than me and his bike was fully loaded. The first part of the freewheel was the best as it was slow motion with the bikes side by side, two grinning jockeys aboard and plenty of banter.

'Put your back into it.'

'Hey, no pedalling.'

Within 20 metres my bike was already a bike length ahead and accelerating. It confirmed that I had packed everything including the kitchen sink.

Mike liked to walk up the steeper hills so he soon dropped back. John looked to have legs that wouldn't tire; he set a brisk pace. I fell back slightly from John but maintained a strong enough pace not to lose him. The thing about riding in a group on the TA was that, in reality, you were really still riding on your own; everyone had their own pace.

Luigi was back from me. The occasional glance back confirmed that he wasn't dropping off.

It was only 27km from Matamata to the start of the Waikato River Trail. The northern trailhead began at Lake Karapiro.

I was in my element on the lightly technical trail. It was family friendly so not very challenging but it had enough changes of elevation and twists to make it interesting.

Luigi and John weren't so impressed and were pleased to break back onto the seal near Arapuni. It was becoming clear to me that most of the riders on this tour were road cyclists. Not mountain bikers.

A couple of young women were messing about in the front yard of a house in Arapuni. Luigi enquired of them as to where a store could be found. They smiled and said there was no store. Strange, as there was certainly a community there, a good number of houses, a population of several hundred.

They invited us in for a drink of water, a friendly introduction to the kicked back village. A tray of marijuana cookies was on the bench awaiting the oven. *That would explain the laidback reception.*

'Did you see that?' hissed Luigi, as our group left the property. 'Dope cookies. And there's no shop in this place. There's something about this town.'

'You may be rushing to conclusions,' I soothed. 'We've only just arrived.'

'No. I know things,' said Luigi, somewhat mysteriously.

I could imagine Luigi as a Catholic priest. Or, a seminarian. A member of a secret order. He had an ethereal quality. Put a dog collar on him and some black robes. He would definitely be a cassock wearer.

The backpackers was just along the road. John decided to continue riding as he said he'd already lost a couple of days due to an injury. He bade adios and powered away.

The landlady at the backpackers was expecting us. She said she had been tracking us. This would make many people paranoid, but this was normal on the TA. Many people were tracking us.

Mike had arrived by this stage. Also, Lou, a large and obviously determined woman. She said she had walked nearly every hill and sometimes looked for a more direct route than that suggested by the official guide.

I had my room booked. A room with a double bed and a set of bunks. There was one other room that had two sets of bunks. There was plenty of room in the yard for tents.

I quickly unloaded my bike and put the bags into my room. I ignored Luigi who was taking a sly peek into my room, noting the bunk beds adjacent to the double.

The landlady was saying that the room with two sets of bunks was all she had left. Mike, Lou and Luigi were considering this: I could see the ruminations playing out in their brains. Bunks and Bunkhouse were not words one wanted to hear on reaching a certain age. Sharing a room, especially a small one with bunks such as this, was something that became less and less appealing as one grew older. Older women tended to become more manlike in their sleeping habits. Burps, snuffling and the occasional fart became part of their sleep repertoire. Plus, of course, the need for a shave in the morning.

'I don't snore,' said Luigi, a little too forcefully.

'Neither,' said Mike.

'Don't think so,' said Lou.

The trio looked doubtfully at one another.

I turned my attention to my room. I quietly departed the scene, and firmly shut the door to my room. I slipped my cleats off and lay back on the bed. *Ah*.

The landlord turned up an hour later. He'd been driving a bus for the local school run. The bus had broken down, which hadn't left him in the best of moods.

Luigi was blissfully unaware of his crankiness. 'How come Arapuni doesn't have a shop?' he asked.

'Because it doesn't,' replied the landlord, somewhat aggressively.

Northern England was where I placed the man's accent. Definitely working-class. From Yorkshire or thereabouts – *a region where complaining was like breathing.*

'It could do with a store,' Luigi ploughed on.

'Well, it doesn't have one,' the landlord replied, folding his arms with some satisfaction.

'Surely someone has wanted to put one in.'

'Many have tried. But they won't allow it.'

'Who won't allow it?'

'The town. The people who run the town.'

'Oh. You mean the council?' said Luigi. There must be rules: Luigi lived by rules – there must be degree and discipline. *People weren't animals.*

'No. The people who make the decisions.'

'And who are they?'

'A few people. The owners of the town.' The landlord smiled enigmatically, and left that hanging.

Luigi nodded and equally smiled back. The smile of someone who had just confirmed a theory. 'Any chance of some food, then?'

As there was no store, the backpackers just happened to have a freezer full of food. If you could call it that. (They would in the north of England). It was all in packages, mostly small cardboard packages. Lasagne, meatballs, shepherd's pie. And quite expensive compared to what it would cost at, say, a store.

A decent meal was proving elusive on the tour. The Covid virus had closed most cafes outside of the main centres. It had also closed many shops. However, that didn't matter in Arapuni: the place with no shops but the amazing backpacker's freezer.

Lou, Mike, Luigi and I contemplated the smorgasbord – we knew the picture on the packet would bear little resemblance to what was inside. Lasagne was the popular choice.

There was a small kitchen cum dining room, it was convivial and certainly cosy. It had a microwave and the basics to help with turning the consumables into food.

Mike had recently cycled in Africa and some Arab countries. Mike did not look like a cyclist but looks could be deceiving in the cycling world; he was no mug. He was also a mine of information when it came to navigation. He showed me how to load the Topo app onto my phone. He then downloaded the GPS trail for the TA and overlaid it onto the Topo map of NZ. You could zoom it in and out with a pinch of your fingers. Enhance a town or swipe to scroll down the length of the country. I was dumbstruck. This was incredible. Life on the tour had suddenly changed. I would know where I was going. Imagine that? No more having to put an ear to the ground – having to look for broken branches – a trail of bread – sniffing age residue off a pile of dung.

Life is beautiful. Modern technology that is actually of use. I had a mount on my bars for the phone, true, but the phone had largely become an ornament – now it could become Command Central.

I hit the bed early. My own room and it was heaven. Next door I could hear sounds of shuffling and bumping. No doubt sorting out who was for which bunk. The three of them. All non-snorers. *Yeah, right.*

I woke in the middle of the night – my bladder needing attention. It was a shared bathroom for those in the bunkrooms. I saw no point in going there and knocking around making noise, trying to find light switches, banging the toilet seat. I headed straight from the door into the open yard.

I'm still in bed, it's cosy, my head is still on the pillow – I sought to maintain mid-sleep momentum. I kept my eyes closed as much as possible – *I was still in bed.* However, midstream I discerned that there was a faint light to my right. I reluctantly opened one eye and peered dimly towards the source. Some kind of luminescence: a dull white light like that from a nest of glow-flies – although this seemed unnatural. I opened the other eye. The soft light was coming from a screen – from an iPad or tablet. And there was the quick glow of a cigarette. The landlady was sitting at a table sucking a fag while scanning her device, at 2am.

Next moment a light from the barn came on, perfectly framing me in the middle of the yard. One of those sensor lights, except it was a little late with its entrance.

I froze, at least my bladder did. I looked again to the glow but there was no movement, no indication that the landlady was watching me. *Was she operating a switch to the security light on the barn?*

I snuck back to my room, with a small intake of guilt, feeling like a thief – caught.

I was first up next morning and into the breakfast room; breakfast was included in the price. There was cereal and toast. The other three TA'ers arrived soon after. They looked a little the worse for wear.

'Last time I'm ever going to share a room,' muttered Luigi. 'I didn't sleep. *He* snored all night.'

He, meaning Mike.

'Mate, it was you that was snoring, believe me,' laughed Mike. Lou rolled her eyes in agreement. I suspected she was also a likely culprit. Lou looked like she had a snore in her. It was a case of Mr Peacock in the library with the candlestick and no one was going to take the rap.

Speaking of peacock. 'Did you fellas get up in the night for a pee?' I enquired.

'Yeah, in the garden,' said Mike. 'And the bloody light came on halfway through.'

'Did you notice anything else?' I asked.

'No.'

'I did,' offered Luigi, pulling up a chair. 'I went into the yard for a leak and the woman of the house was sitting on her porch watching. Smoking a ciggy and playing on her computer. Then the light came on.'

'I reckon she has a switch for that barn light,' I said. 'She probably has a camera set up and films all the fellas that go out for a pee. Your knob is now on record.'

'Good luck to her,' coughed Luigi. 'This town is weird. I reckon the reason there's no shops here is because the place is run by gangsters. They come here to hide out away from the law.'

I had to agree that there was a funny vibe to the place.

Small town NZ.

Arapuni to Pureora

25km sealed road, 28km dirt and gravel, 50km gravel cycleway

I beat Mike in a couple of early freewheel contests before the group split due to people's varying pace. Lou dropped back early. Mike next. Luigi was steady on the hills and climbed well. I was quickest downhill and slightly faster than the others on the flats.

It was another nice day for cycling. Cool, dry and no wind.

At 20km we three guys regrouped for the Waikato River Trail run through to Mangakino. Lou was nowhere to be seen. As was her way, she had begun walking at the first hill. Slow but steady. The tortoise and the hare.

Mike, Luigi and I had little hair amongst us. 'Hair is for girls,' my dad used to say. Baldness wasn't the only common denominator amongst us: we discovered that we were all from Whangārei – some coincidence eh. Whangārei was dairy farming country – but there was no cream rising to the top here: we weren't athletes, in the traditional sense. But we had fortitude. Perhaps not as much as a girl named Lou.

The river trail was lovely. Well-groomed and one of the most well used trails in the NZ network. I was in my element on the trail and moved ahead of the others.

Mangakino was perfectly placed at 54km from Arapuni. A couple of cafes and a bakery. The TA was a boon for little towns like this. To be fair, Mangakino looked not much bigger than Arapuni, yet it had a multitude of shops, including a supermarket. It was a regular stop off for cyclists doing the Waikato trails and for those going on to do the Timber Trail.

We were going to need to feed as the next 40km was all uphill – 600 metres of uphill.

The climb gradually steepened as we got into it. The native bush was thick either side of the road – there was a series of damns along the river. Very little traffic. Slow going for motorists with many tight corners.

There was little talk amongst our trio; small thoughts and steady breathing. The road tightened. I peeled out the guidebook: 'When the road seems to end, veer left down the hill and you'll reach a narrow wire bridge over the Mangakino Stream.'

The Pureora Forest had begun. So too did some light but steady rain. The 'narrow wire bridge' meant bags off the bike and carried over. The bike was then stood on its back wheel and wheeled across. This would become the method for crossing many bridges in the coming days.

I had crossed a lot of bush bridges in my youth. The Blockhouse Bay Boys Brigade was big on the great outdoors and I had been a keen member. The Waitakeres and the Kahurangi National Park had provided a lot of adventures. Fording rivers was part of tramping in NZ. Bridges were '*luxury*' – in your best Monty Python voice. Three-wire bridges could be terrifying – especially with some dickhead bouncing on the other end. One wire for each hand and a bottom wire for your feet. Character building.

I contemplated this bridge into the Pureora Forest – a loose term for the construction; you wouldn't want to be afraid of heights. It was basically a three-wire bridge with a rotted strip of plywood wide down the middle. *'Luxury, rotting wood – in my day';* classic for Pythonites.

The ply was wide enough to place one foot at a time. Definitely one person at a time and you needed regular stops to allow the bridge to cease swaying so you could continue the crossing. I briefly considered being the 'dickhead' and bouncing the bridge. However, I didn't really yet know the fellas I was with – and they were bigger than me.

The next 15km was all walking for the three intrepid Whangārei travellers.

Thick bush, 4WD drive and single track. I lost one of my flags somewhere in the bush – the silver fern one. It must have snagged on a low branch. Homer was strangely silent. He was a long way from home, a long way from Marge.

Near the base of Mt Titiraupenga, a monument had been placed on the trail, marking the centre of the North Island. It felt like it, to me. 'The centre of the North Island' – a seemingly bland statement. But, oh no, not without controversy.

If you travelled through the Waikato and into the King Country, several places along the way claimed to be at the very centre. Just north of Matamata, the tiny town of Waharoa proposed having a plaque engraved: "Middle of North Island. Waharoa. You are Here."

Land Information NZ Chief Topographer, John Spittal, said there was no exact centre of the North Island and it was such an uneven shape that there was no practical centre. He reckoned there were several ways to work out a mid-point, but each gave a different location.

Hamilton LINZ went scientific and used latitude and longitude. It came up with Horahora, a small farming community just south of Cambridge, as the middle. Ironically, Horahora made no claim to it.

Transit NZ estimated the midway distance between Cape Reinga and Wellington, via SH27, would be about 3km on the Tirau side of Hinuera.

I read the origins of the obelisk in front of me. Its location was the work of a local surveyor – he took some cardboard and cut out the shape of the North Island and found the point where it balanced on a pin.

Perfect, I grinned. *It was done by weight.*

Light rain was falling as the lads battled along. The last 8km were downhill on a rocky forestry road. I had stubbornly been maintaining high tyre pressures but even that was not enough to save my rear tyre – there were a lot of sharp rocks. It loudly blew with only a couple of km's to go to the Pureora cabins. I had been travelling quicker than was advisable for the state of the trail, but I wanted to get to the cabins early and see if I could nab one. I was sure the blown tube would only be a minor inconvenience – I could change a tube in minutes.

However, the 50/50 rule was still at play in my life. I had had a 50 percent chance of grabbing the right sort of tube off the shelf in the bike shop. Without checking, I bought a tube with a Schrader valve. It should have been one with a Presta valve.

It wouldn't work in my wheel. The valve was too large to go through the hole in the rim. I also noticed, while waiting for the others, that the tyre had a worrying split in it. The upside of running a high pressure was that the tyre would roll faster. The downside was that if you got a puncture it was more likely to be catastrophic. I really needed a new tyre too.

Luigi had a puncture repair kit.

'This isn't some Italian knock off kit, is it?' I asked, looking dubious about its quality. *Still, beggars can't be choosers.*

'Not that I'm aware,' replied Luigi. 'But it could be.' He laughed. 'Did you ever read the smallest Italian book?'

'Not that I'm aware,' I said, trying to get a nice square of glue on the tube, while sheltering it from the rain.

'Italian war heroes,' chuckled Luigi.

Mike and Luigi decided to peddle ahead to the Pureora campground. *And first dibs at any cabins*, as I put the wheel back together. I pumped air into the tyre. Nothing. I pumped more air into the tyre. Nothing. It didn't inflate. The patch had lifted immediately.

Bloody Italians. I loved Valentino Rossi but Italy had its shortfalls. It wasn't known for the reliability of its vehicles. Incredible cars like Ferrari and Lamborghini. Motorcycles like Ducati and MotoGuzzi. But an Italian machine was a fickle beast. Italian engineering left a lot to be desired.

Mama Mia.

The Kopiko Aotearoa happened to be running simultaneously with the TA. The KA was a bike packing trip (also invented by the Kennett brothers) from Cape Egmont to East Cape, or vice versa. The Timber Trail was the only spot where the two rides intersected. It just so happened that a small group of KA'ers were passing through just then, much to my good fortune. One of them had a couple of spare 29er tubes. He gave one to me, with the words: 'You can do the same to someone further down the line.' *Sweet.*

Also passing by was a local with a flatdeck ute. He offered me a ride down the last couple of k's to the camp. I placed my bike on the back and off we went, even managing to overtake Mike and Luigi with a few hundred metres to go.

Great. Still a chance to get in for a cabin.

Alas, no. They were all taken. Well, not all. But under level 2 Covid restrictions, the managers were only letting out every second cabin; so as to keep space between. Despite all the occupants intermingling with one another – sharing their breath, spittle and whatever other juices were flowing.

I stood with my hands on my hips. The rain was still falling – it was light, but had been constant since we entered the Pureora Forest.

Righto, onwards. First duty was to tend to my steed and get the wheel back together. Second was to find a tent spot. Might as well set up while still in my wet gear, besides it was getting late.

Luigi was also breaking out his tent, which, strangely enough, was the same brand as mine – Big Agnes. Although, as Luigi pointed out, his was the biking version and mine was the hiking version – not quite as good for bike packing.

Mike had a tent he had never used. It was new and he wanted to keep it that way. He stood on the deck, out of the rain, soberly watching Luigi and I, on our knees, unpacking tour tents. He desperately wanted an alternative – he was reticent to erect his pup.

Just then Lou appeared. Not appeared in the puff of smoke sense, but something close. She was in dry clothes and had the blush of someone recently showered. Lou climbed the steps to the deck and joined Mike.

They gazed down at their fellow travellers. A KA'er, Kate, was also setting up a tent. Hers was also brand new though unlike Mike, Kate wanted to test it. She had alternative accommodation available in a cabin but she was hardy. *True spunk.*

Luigi noticed that he was being watched. He rose slowly to his feet and turned to address Lou: 'How is it possible,' he enquired, with a hint of annoyance, 'That you are here before us? Did you pass us?'

We had clearly left her behind, that very morning, on the first hill.

'No, I stayed on the road, on Highway 30,' she replied, rising on her toes and sweeping her arms wide, palms up. 'It seemed like a good option.' She lowered her feet and her arms. 'I read the guide and it didn't sound good.' Lou squinted at Luigi. 'How was that narrow wire bridge?'

Luigi squinted back and pursed his lips. 'Narrow,' he said. He raised his eyebrows and looked meaningfully at Lou. 'It was a squeeze. Very tight.'

'Where are you staying?' enquired Mike, turning to Lou – hope lightly building in his eyes.

'I got the last cabin.'

'How big is it?' asked Mike, hope becoming a beacon.

'Oh, it's big. Why, would you like to share?'

'Yes, please,' said Mike, his face radiant.

They shuffled off together, as happy as pigs in shit.

Luigi and I saw to our tents and headed for the showers – which were fantastic: plenty of force and hot.

A bunch of KA'ers were in the other cabins. We introduced ourselves. Space was found on the deck for our bikes and it was most convivial. The deck was chocka with hanging gear and bikes.

There was much oohing and aahing at the different Surly models on the deck. Names like Karate Monkey, Krampus, Ogre, Pugsley and Straggler. I suddenly found myself in the midst of a Surly lovefest.

The riders touched each other's bikes with affection, clucking and purring in the back of their throats. I felt a little sick coming into the back of *my* throat. I rode a Giant; I was excluded from the conversation. *Fine by me*, I reckoned, and moved away from the icky Surly love.

Mike and Lou reappeared. They had Surlys.

Must have heard the strange Surly incantations. I slid further away from the group.

The cyclists in the cabin near Luigi and I were very friendly and offered the use of their kitchen. I discovered that Kate and I knew someone in common – not an unusual occurrence in NZ. My brother-in-law, Murray, was good mates with Kate. Kate bantered that she wouldn't tell Murray that she found me blubbing in the bathroom. Wanting to go home to momma. Whatever.

I had a dehydrated meal that just needed boiling water. It was roast chicken and mashed potato. *Incredible*, I pondered, while trying to read the directions. How could you possibly think the dried mix inside the foil bag could turn into roast chicken?

There was a bag within the bag. This contained the mashed potato. There was spillage on the floor of the cabin but I wasn't convinced that it was from me. I was incriminated by being on the scene – I did my best to clean it up, or at least to use my shoe to sweep it somewhere that the sun didn't shine.

The roast chicken was delicious. The mashed spud was nearly perfect – could have just done with a little butter.

Luigi had crackers and slices of salami for his dinner.

He didn't appear to be that well organised, I noted. He might give me the 'holier than thou' attitude but who was eating the roast chicken, eh? *It was probably Luigi's crackers spilt on the floor.*

Lou and Mike were nowhere to be seen.

It had been a huge day and bed was calling. Besides, Luigi and I didn't have anywhere to hang out, with dark having fallen and a steady drizzle coming down.

Timber Trail to Taumaranui

70km single track, 20km gravel, 14km seal

It seemed to take forever to pack. The light rain falling didn't make it easy. The trick was to keep the water outside the tent. It was no fun packing a wet tent but it had to be done.

Out here on the steppes of Mongolia. The wilds. *Only a yak for company. Ee ba gum.* A little exaggeration.

I made tea for Luigi and myself and cooked porridge on the deck by the bathroom. My little Trangia stove was a winner: that's why I lugged that bottle of meths around; *it wasn't only for drinking.*

The Timber Trail was heavily forested at its beginning. The drizzly rain only just penetrated the tree cover. It fell as intermittent large drops. A couple of kilometres in and my tyre blew with gusto. To be more exact, the tube blew – at the split in the tyre.

I had no more tubes. Luigi's tube repair kit had been buried in the Italian war heroes cemetery – *there was plenty of room.* I had to concede that it probably wasn't an Italian tyre repair kit; *but someone had to take the rap.* I reflected that I should have packed a repair kit but usually a spare tube was enough backup.

I decided I would walk my bike back to where Pureora joined Highway 30 and hitch a ride to Taumaranui to buy a tyre and tubes.

Luigi didn't like that idea. He generously offered up his only spare tube. That would leave the two of us with no spare tubes. It was a magnanimous offer. The truth was that Luigi didn't want to cycle alone. He operated best with a wingman.

The tube proved to be too wide for my wheel, in theory. I noted that it was also too wide for Luigi's. Gradually I was learning more about *Wing Commander Herr Luigi*. He wasn't as well prepared as he appeared. Sure, he could talk knowledgably of Surly legendary exploits – the merits of one Aunt Agnes tent over another – but there was a bumbling, doltish aspect to his overall package. He wasn't quite the finished product.

Perhaps this wingman job was more of a batman job, I wondered. Not the Robin and Batman show but the Biggles and batman one. The batman who was servant to a commissioned officer in the RAF in WW2.

I cut a section out of my old tube and used it as a sleeve between the new tube and the split in the tyre. A packer. The new tube was a little large but with careful stuffing it fitted inside the tyre and was inflated – not to 70lbs – more like 30.

'You shouldn't have cut that tube,' said Luigi, pointing at the old tube in my hand. 'You can tie a knot in a tube, where the hole is, and that will stop it leaking.'

I looked dubiously at Luigi. 'Have you been having flashbacks of the McIver series?'

'No, I've seen it on YouTube,' said Luigi, with authority. 'You tie a knot where the leak is and it's as good as new.'

I contemplated this nugget of information. 'Surely you would have to tie a knot on either side of the hole.' I am nothing if not a practical man. Things had to make sense to me. There was a mountain of information out there and with the advent of forums like, Facebook, I suspected the mountain was mostly Mt Misinformation.

'Well, I've seen it,' said Luigi, not quite so boldly.

'Okay, when you get a flatty, we will tie a knot in it,' I replied, with satisfaction. 'Seems like we don't actually need any spare tubes then.'

Luigi frowned and began pulling his gloves back on.

The tube cum packer bulged a little through the split in my tyre but appeared to be holding.

We had lost an hour messing about with the tyre. However, we caught up with Mike in surprisingly quick time. He was struggling with the wet conditions as his tyres were more road orientated with their tread pattern. The track was proving a little slick for them.

The gradient was gentle but firm, like a nun. It was 13km to the top of the climb and after that, mostly flat and downhill. The sound of kaka screeched through the lower slopes. Further up, it was tui and kereru.

'Where's Lou?' asked Luigi.

'She left early, before light,' replied Mike. 'She's slow so needs a full day.'

The Timber Trail Lodge was the planned oasis. It was at the midway point on the trail and was offering a pizza and drink for $10 to TA riders. It took us four hours to get there. A steady 5kph on our carthorses. We passed several KA riders going the other way, who all seemed full of good cheer and were noticeably travelling faster than us – lightly packed and on the move. The KA was only a 1000km ride. More of a splash and dash than the TA. However, its course was tougher. This was its second year.

The Timber Trail Lodge had bicycle tubes for sale. With Presta valves. The price was high, but when you're marooned on a desert island and a bottle of rum washes up, you don't bemoan the fact that there's no ice.

I bought two tubes and gave one to Luigi: 'I know you don't need it, with your knot trick and all.'

'Hey, it works,' said Luigi, only a little affronted.

Lou wasn't at the lodge but the KA crew from the past night was. They were travelling in the vice versa direction to the other KA'ers that we had met. They joined us on the wide deck.

Kate was in full cheer. She was one of those healthy, outdoor girls – all plaits and bounce. 'Just been talking on the phone to Murray,' said Kate. 'He said that we need to spend less time sitting about and more time in the saddle. Cheeky bugger, eh? So how are you holding up?'

'Mid-afternoon my knees are screaming children,' I answered. 'Other than that, I feel fine.'

Kate and her crew finished their meal, mounted up and headed back to the Timber Trail.

Luigi and I settled into chairs facing the hills. The pizza and drink were a fine concept. There were no milkshakes available, however. That could be worked on. Our pizzas arrived.

'What is the name for the pizza featuring the colours of the Italian flag?' asked Luigi. 'The tricolour.'

'You weren't a schoolteacher, were you?' I asked.

Luigi wasn't going to be distracted: 'The pizza is called a Margherita. And what food makes each colour?'

'Red, tomato, obviously,' I said. 'Green, basil.'

Luigi looked a little surprised that I would know this vegetable.

'And the white is cheese.'

'Yes, but what cheese?'

'Mozzarella,' I said, with quiet satisfaction. Sometimes my brain did work.

'What animal does mozzarella come from?'

Doh, said my brain. *Had to be a catch.* 'A cow.'

'No,' said Luigi, a kind tone to his voice.

Kind, but slightly condescending, I thought.

'Clue. It is a farm animal.'

'A pig.'

'No.'

'A goat. No, that would be feta.'

We spied Mike coming up the path below the lodge. Pushing his bike. The lodge deck offered a magnificent view over the adjacent valley. A first-rate platform to sit with a beer and a .308 and pot deer coming out on the far hill.

'A deer.'

'No.'

Mike was red in the face and breathing heavily as he slumped into the chair opposite. He ordered two pizzas from the waiter. Luigi and I ordered another one, to split.

Mike explained that he was struggling with fading brakes. The Surly brake system was cable operated as opposed to the hydraulics of most modern bikes. It made sense as Surly was built to be taken off the beaten track. It had to be simple and easy to repair. It was the bike that Bear Grylls would select to take into the Andes, or Amazon. It was rugged and you could repair a cable operated brake system using vines and Orangutang bottom.

I went and made a quick inspection of the brake pads on Mike's Surly. They were very low. Nearly through to the metal. And you know what would happen then? Bone on bone, with no cartilage. Then arthritis, followed by lack of movement. And night aches.

We left Mike to his pizza. It was time for us to forge ahead. Mike was in for a long day. He was now having to walk down the hills to go with his walking up the hills. This left him with little actual cycling time. A long day but a lovely trail to walk. It was also part of the Te Araroa Trail, so it was well walked.

I took it easy on the downhill stretches to be gentle on the split tyre. I used the brakes more than I wished. I preferred to give the Giant its head: let it run. But not this day: carrying all that weight, especially with the load over the front wheel, meant that on gravel or loose dirt, the tyres would occasionally lose purchase as they were overwhelmed. The front wheel would tuck slightly and I was surprised how quickly I would catch these slides. Built into me from my dirt bike riding days I guess. It was good that I caught these slides as the next stage would be a full folding of the front end and over the bars flying, a-la-Superman. This could result in broken body bits or dental work. Technical name: *frontal Barlotomy*, I named it.

The trick to any off-road downhill, on any bike, was to stand up. To let the bike move under the rider. Bend the knees slightly, elbows wide, bum back and let the bike absorb the bumps while the body flowed over them.

Luigi wouldn't stand on his pedals. He complained bitterly about the bumps in the track and was looking forward to the seal. I encouraged him to try standing. It could change his life. Luigi reckoned he got cramp in his left calf if he tried standing.

Luigi, with his mismatched socks, fluro orange top and his bug-eyed goggles, was quite a sight. The convex lenses made Luigi look like a giant fly.

I cycled closer to Luigi. I tried again: 'Mozzarella comes from a horse.'

'No.'

The Timber Trail finished at the Ongarue Spiral. The spiral was spectacular. An ingenious way to get a timber tram down a steep section. It comprised a low-level bridge, a deep cutting, a curved tunnel, an over-bridge and a complete circle of the track.

The track didn't really finish there, but it felt like it should. It kept going and going for what seemed like ages, but was only in fact, another 10km to the village of Ongarue. Ongarue was at the junction of Highway 4 and a couple of other roads. It was once a thriving centre. Now it was a derelict gathering of slums. Barns, sheds and houses built with native timber. All now, sadly, sagging and fading like old drag queens. Once bright and pouty, now down-mouthed and sombre.

The Ongarue Rugby Club, a grand old wooden building, was the exemplar. It was rotting in all its glory beside what was once a rugby field.

The word was that people had tried to buy it, to turn it into a backpackers, but it wasn't for sale. The locals didn't want change. Ongarue was one up on Arapuni, though, it had a store. The Ongarue Store.

Darkness was creeping in. It was 24km on gravel to Taumaranui, or 24km on seal on Highway 4.

'Moose,' I said.

'No.'

'A farm animal?'

'Yes. A farm animal in Italy.'

'Donkey.'

'No.'

We opted for a sprint on the seal in an effort to beat the dark. But sunset, along with sunrise, was one of the most dangerous times to ride a bicycle. Especially on the open road with Kiwi drivers in their jalopies, their throttle feet nailed to the floor.

This was our first riding together where lights were required. I dug around in a pannier and came up with a headlight. It was in two pieces having fallen apart due to its quality; lack of. Lights were usually measured in units of lumens – my light was more in the candle strength category. My taillight was permanently mounted and had the flicker feature, however it too was feeble – more an annoyance than a serious take notice light.

'What do you have in the light department?' I asked.

'You mean, what don't I have in the way of lights,' replied Luigi, wickedly. With an incandescent flourish, he pulled two compact lights from his bar bag: one with a red lens and the other with a white. He held aloft the red one. 'I call this, Godzilla.'

'And why?'

'You will see.' Luigi looked condescendingly at the light in my hand, which was still in two pieces. 'Is that thing worth even carrying?'

'You never know when you might need it,' I said, loosely inspecting it. Wondering if there was a possibility it would ever be needed; or would work when required.

'You won't be able to lead with that, thing,' said Luigi, with a haughty tone. 'I will lead, you ride tail-end-Charley. Even your taillight isn't up to it, but beggars can't be choosers.'

I could make no argument; I dearly wanted to.

Luigi switched on Godzilla.

(I caught a flash of it in a cornea and went down. Frothing at the mouth and blood squirting from my ears.) *Geez man*, I panicked...*that didn't happen but it definitely could happen.* So much brightness emanating from such a small device. Godzilla was bright enough to peel paint from a billboard.

'Is that thing legal?' I enquired, genuinely distressed. We decided that my job, as wingman (now tailman), was to follow Luigi and yell whenever a truck was coming from behind.

'I don't know,' said Luigi, chuckling. 'I was using Godzilla in a group, a while back, and this guy got really angry and tried to attack me. But he couldn't see me as he was partially blinded.' Luigi guffawed, 'He said he was an epileptic.'

Hilarious. I suffered migraines. Usually brought on by bright light. *Perfect.*

I immediately dropped back behind Luigi – about one km back. Still, the red light bounced off the surrounding hills. Incredible.

Luigi pulled up at the roadside and waited for me. 'I lost you.'

'No. I dropped back. I'm trying to save my eyesight. I may need it in the future.'

Luigi laughed. 'It's that bright?'

'Brighter than that. It can't be legal.'

'I can charge it with a USB cable. Brilliant.' Luigi was well pleased with it.

I was less enthusiastic. 'It could bring down a plane. I can't believe that thing's legal.'

Luigi gave me an uncharitable glance: 'See if you can keep up,' he said, pedalling away.

Ha. Easy for him to say. Flashing his Godzilla terror around the country.

I stayed slightly closer to Luigi's tail. I hugged the white line trying to stay to the left of the light's beam. I also had to keep looking over my shoulder for any oncoming truck and trailer units. Then yell 'truck.'

Halfway to Taumaranui, a station wagon slowed and pulled alongside. A man was leaning out the passenger window.

'So long, suckers!' he yelled. It was Mike. The owner of the motel we were booked into, had gone to pick him up. Mike had done well to make it to Ongarue before total nightfall. He had had some scary moments sliding down the Timber Trail, legs out like outriggers, shoes dragging for purchase.

'Later alligator,' yelled Mike, as they sped away to Taumaranui.

I closed the gap to Luigi. 'Mozzarella. Alligator,' I called.

'Predictable. No'

'Guinea pig.'

'Now you're being silly.'

We made the motel at 9pm. Darkness had fallen.

And who should be there to greet us, but Lou. Showered and looking fresh. She even had had time to do her laundry. Bryan, the motel owner, had apparently run to Ongarue for her, too.

A girl named Lou… from Ongarue, I sang to myself, as I climbed the stairs to my room.

The motel was $100 for a room and immaculate. It was hard to describe the feeling I had, as I looked into my room. A king-sized bed with towels placed on the end of it. A table. A kitchenette. A large bathroom with more fluffy towels. Soaps, shampoos, smelly tubes. I felt that same feeling you had when canoodled by a large breasted woman of great bouquet.

Bryan said the RSA was keeping its kitchen open but we must go immediately, no time to shower. A fine act of generosity. Mike and Lou were showered. Luigi and I didn't mind – we were hungry.

'Mike,' I said, as we were seated. 'Where does mozzarella come from?'

'Buffalo,' replied Mike.

Luigi smiled sweetly.

'Wanker,' I said.

PART TWO

The Little Things

Taumaranui

Day off

Heavy rain on the window greeted me as I pulled back the curtain in the motel room. It was still dark. I headed back to bed, the king-size bed.

You could have been forgiven for thinking that the room had been the scene of a crime. A bad one, involving a tramper and a weather incident – like a hurricane. A tent was hanging off a curtain hook. The tent fly was flung over another hook. Sleeping bag from yet another hook. And clothes all about, on chairs, desk and the bench.

I was drying my camping gear.

I texted Luigi. 'Hey, my legs have stopped working. My knees are shot. Having a day off. Going to stay here another night.'

Luigi replied shortly. 'In full agreement. Body battery needs recharging.'

Wimp, I thought.

Mike also took the day out to get his brakes looked at. Lou decided to stop too. The rain was solid and the forecast was better for the next day.

I went down to the office and enquired of Bryan, the motel owner, as to where a bike shop might be.

'What do you need?' asked Bryan.

'I've split a tyre so I need one of those.'

'What size?'

'29er.'

Bryan reached down behind the counter and came up with a tyre. Slightly dusty, but a 29-inch tyre. 'Can give you this for 90 bucks.'

I was dubious.

'There's no bicycle shop in Taumaranui,' said Bryan, somewhat pompously. 'There's a motorbike shop. This is the tyres they sell there.'

'Oh,' I said. 'Okay.' I preferred the idea of buying from a shop – of having a choice. 'Good to know.'

'You won't find better than this.'

'Mike needs some brakes, too, so I'll go with him for a bit.' I was losing my appetite for this conversation.

'What sort of brakes is he running?' asked Bryan, ducking down again behind the counter and coming up with another dusty pack. 'I have these Shimano pads.'

'No, he's running a Surly.'

'These should fit,' said Bryan.

'No, they're different.'

'The problem won't be with his pads,' said Bryan, with authority.

Here we go, I thought. He runs a great motel. However, Brian's alter ego was that he was another one of the WGA brigade. (World's Great Authority).

'I had a look at them,' I continued. 'The pads are worn through.'

'I doubt it,' said Bryan, defensively.

'Surly make their own system,' I said, patiently; it was too early for the blood to rise. 'It's a cable operated system, not hydraulic. A good idea, as you can probably fix them if you're stuck out in the boonies.'

'What's wrong with hydraulic?' said Bryan. 'I've never had trouble with hydraulic.'

'Well, you do need gear with hydraulic. To bleed them. They can be tricky.'

'Ha,' said Bryan, a blush rising to his face. 'I just squeeze them. That's how you bleed them.'

'Anyways,' I said, trying to steer the conversation back to safe ground. 'It's the brake pads that need replacing. Worn out.'

'You don't run out of pads.'

'You've never used up a set of pads?' I asked, a small smile creeping onto my face. It looked like this fella wasn't going to let it go. My blood began stirring.

'Never,' said Bryan boldly. 'Never run out of brakes.'

'Perhaps we do a different type of riding to each other,' I offered, kindly. Okay, maybe laced with a small spread of sarcasm. The Kiwi way. Hard not to, when a WGA makes its appearance.

'I've done every sort of riding,' stated Bryan. 'Done it all. Never used up any brakes.'

'How do you not use up brakes. What if you're riding steep tracks for hours?'

'I don't brake,' said Bryan, emphatically, folding his arms. 'I just go fast. No braking.'

Amazing how quickly you can go from being a good bloke to a dork.

'Could you recommend a café?' I asked, cheerfully.

I hovered on the office doorstep. Should I ask Bryan whether he knew which animal mozzarella came from? But what if he said, buffalo?

Luigi was up and also looking for breakfast.

'Guess I pissed Bryan off,' I said, as we set to walking to the main street. 'Didn't buy his tyre off him.'

'Ah, yes, me too,' confessed Luigi, grinning. 'I asked him about doing the Bridge to Nowhere track.' Luigi chuckled. 'Bryan said, "You can't do it in this weather." So, I asked him if he'd done the TA. A perfectly innocent question. Well, he wasn't happy, was he?'

Luigi smiled and changed his voice: "I don't have time for that. I have a motel to run."

'And he does run a good one,' I chuckled. 'It's just that ego thing. Having to prove you are the big dog.'

'I don't give a fuck what they think,' said Luigi, somewhat fiercely.

We found breakfast at a café and also found John, the older chap who'd been with us from Matamata. Funny how you kept bumping into fellow TA'ers despite people cycling at different paces.

John said he had also cycled with JB, back when we were in Northland. It was good to know JB was still out there. John said it had been near Poutu that he came across JB, who had suggested they ride together. He said JB only lasted one hill and then went and lay down by the side of the road.

John had a full knee replacement surgery a year before and said it was fantastic. You wouldn't have known he'd been under the knife. He was as strong as an ox – or a buffalo.

I bought a cheap tyre from the motorcycle shop. I decided not to fit it but to stay with my current tyre with the split in it. The split hadn't gotten worse and although it was bulging through the tear, it looked okay. The cheapie would be a reserve parachute.

Mike found some brake pads at the motorcycle shop. Amazing. On a back shelf they had a set of Surly brake pads.

It was nice to have a day off. It was also nice to walk the streets of a NZ town with no undies on. To swing free – very liberating. When you pack light you have to forgo some of the items usually considered essential.

There were worse places to live than Taumaranui, I contemplated. Such as Matamata. Now that was a pretentious place. Overpriced food and accommodation. A characterless farm town in the middle of nowhere that didn't even have a hill, let alone a mountain to give it some feel. Made famous by a film featuring hairy-footed hobbits. It's moment of glory. Really it was just a wet shithole.

Taumaranui didn't suffer from a shortage of rain. But it had hills and even mountains surrounding it. And a mighty river. It had tons of character. Although, it did have a brooding presence as well – slightly sinister. Probably due to the cloud that hung low over the town at every opportunity.

Give me character over bland, flat shithole any day, I reckoned.

However, Taumaranui was doing it hard. Many of the shops were closed, especially up the side streets. Formerly there had been an entrepreneurial air to the town. There were some classic shops: Dr Jekyll's Emporium being one example. Now closed, with plywood covering its opening. And who would have thought Taumaranui would have the best fish and chip shop in NZ? It wasn't even on the coast. But I found it. Fresh deliveries every day. Kina in pottles. Mussels. Creamy paua. Raw fish. I ordered some battered snapper. The owner gave me some smoked salmon wings to sample while I waited. For free. Delicious. *Who knew salmon had wings? Who knew buffalo made mozzarella?*

The day went by quickly and was a great recharge for the mind, body and soul. It also gave time for a little planning. I phoned Whanganui River Adventures for advice on the state of the tracks leading to the Bridge to Nowhere. The very enthusiastic woman, Agatha, on the phone, said it would be fine as some work was being done on the tracks. But it would be slippery. (She said a lot of things, which I missed – I had gone back to the motel for a sleep and she was still talking when I picked up the phone some hours later.) Ok, bit of exaggeration, but Agatha did like to talk.

Luigi, Mike, Lou and I met for dinner at the RSA, again. I found it had lasagne on the menu. If any place could make lasagne, this would be the one. Unfortunately, they had run out.

The conversation turned to the following day and thoughts on riding into the remote depths of the Whanganui River. The other three had had a long chat with Bryan that afternoon and he had advised strongly against it. He said it would be too dangerous with the rain. Wouldn't be passable. I said that I was still keen on doing it. These pieces of the TA were the ones that interested me most. The difficult bits.

'Who's going to tell Bryan?' asked Luigi.

'You,' I said.

Taumaranui to Whakahoro

15km sealed road, 52km gravel

'I've been thinking on it, and I've worked it out,' said Luigi, as we readied our bikes in the half-light of morning. 'Lou has either got an engine in her bike,' he said, leaning delightedly towards me. 'Or she's a witch.'

'You reckon?'

'Yeah, that's how she gets ahead.'

'That would explain the broomstick.'

'Exactly.'

Mike and Lou had decided to heed Bryan's advice. They were going to stay on the highway and bypass the Bridge to Nowhere section. A big call as it was a significant piece of the tour they would miss. It was called the Bridge to Nowhere. *How cool was that?* I was not going to miss it for the world. It was the only piece of the TA that was on my bucket list.

Luigi was torn both ways. He wanted to do it as it was, out there. Held a strong flavour of adventure. However, he didn't like the off-road sections. He favoured the tarmac – hard and fast. But, he didn't want to lose his new wingman.

(He was going to go into the Heart of Darkness with Captain Willard. Take a gunboat upriver, through the Vietcong waters to hunt down and slaughter the traitor Kurtz; little did Luigi know, but *Apocalypse Now* was my favourite movie.)

Luigi liked orderliness. He liked orthodoxy to be his friendly monkey – his sane friendly monkey. He didn't know me. Didn't know what I was capable of. Didn't know how I would act when deep into a fold in the Whanganui River valley. Didn't know if I would tear a mud-streaked strip from my shirt and wind it about my head. Blacken my face with river mud and strap a knife to my side.

Luigi was in a funk. But God, he needed a wingman. The dilemma.

Mike was too slow. Lou would disappear in a puff of smoke. His choices were limited. Luigi breathed deeply and resignedly followed me into the motel office.

'We're going to do the Bridge to Nowhere,' I said brightly, to Bryan, thanking him for the stay, and saying what a great motel he ran.

Luigi didn't say anything. Bryan didn't say anything – he appeared to have sucked a lemon.

It looked like I had made the decision for us.

We pushed our bikes out onto the street. Luigi paused. 'You know that we are now the Lanterne Rouge?'

'The what?' I asked.

'Where do you think we are coming in the TA? What position?'

'We would have to be close to last,' I said, going through my awkward form of the pole vault to get aboard my bike.

'The Lanterne Rouge is the last rider in the Tour de France,' said Luigi. 'It's an honour. We are the Lanterne Rouge of the TA.' Luigi looked well pleased.

I took a moment to let this sink in. 'I've never competed to come last,' I said.

'Exactly. This is a beautiful thing. A great moment. The Lanterne Rouge.' Luigi folded his arms, straightened his shoulders and beamed at me.

I didn't say anything. What could you say? I was clearly cycling with an idiot – who *celebrates losing?*

We gained separation early into the ride – which was a good thing. The RSA meal, the evening before, had affected us both. We hadn't had rich food for a while, and it was probably the dessert that got us. I had needed three visits to the WC that morning. Luigi two. But, we both still had wind. We tooted our way merrily up the valley.

It was a misty morning. The rain had ceased but the atmosphere was dank and heavy, there was a wet cloak hanging about them; the land was a giant shammy.

The first two hours were solid climbing. The seal turned to gravel. I was having my most enjoyable day so far. The Scottish genes loved it when it turned rugged. The Whanganui River flowed below us in all its majestic muddiness.

There were slips at many of the corners from the previous day's rain. The cliffs shed endlessly providing plenty of work for the road crews. The downhills were great fun with lines to be picked between the rocks and ruts. Braking and sliding; so much fun. For Luigi, not so much fun.

Certainly a lot more interesting than ploughing a furrow down the Hauraki Rail Trail or grinding sand along 90 Mile Beach. This was what the TA was about. I was a happy little pig in mud.

We found ourselves at the Blue Duck Inn, after six hours in the saddle. A jetboat had been booked for the following day due to the forecast of treacherous riding. But it had proved to be okay and we made better time than expected. Slippery but fun riding. If we had left earlier we could have caught the jetboat that afternoon.

Should we press on and camp, or have a feed and stay at the Blue Duck cabins? The soft option won, although at $100 for a cabin, basically a plywood box with some bunks, it wasn't cheap. The beauty of a captive market.

I took the top cabin. Luigi the next one down a level. It was lovely. Another magnificent view across hills.

Staying at the Blue Duck cabins turned the Whanganui River stretch of the TA into a three-dayer. Most riders did it in two. Some, in one. It did work out well schedule wise, though, as we would arrive in Whanganui on Sunday evening and get our bikes seen to on Monday morning. We settled in happily with high anticipation for the morrow.

Whakahoro to Pipiriki

10km farm track, 63km single track, 32km jetboat

'Have you read this?' asked Luigi, thrusting the TA guide under my nose.

Note: The Kaiwhakauka Track and Mangapurua Track are both too rough for heavily laden touring bikes – this according to the TA Official Guide.

'Yes. And no,' I replied.

We had tour bikes loaded and ready to go by 7am. It was a leaden sky but it wasn't raining.

'We have heavily laden touring bikes,' said Luigi. 'We should have gone round with Mike and Lou.'

'Perhaps. But we didn't, and here we are. And we have a jetboat booked for four o'clock.' There was some steely satisfaction in my voice. 'Come on, it can't be that bad. We can always walk it.'

I poked a leg over my bike and settled onto the saddle – what I loosely called, my pole vault mount. It wasn't a conventional swing of the leg. Not the usual style one applied when mounting a bicycle, or motorbike, or a horse. More of a straight leg out and spear it over from the side. My hips weren't so flexible anymore and being short in the leg, although tall in the body, I could no longer flex so well. Plus, the flagpole would catch my foot.

The Mountains to Sea trail commenced just down from the Blue Duck. Initially it was a 4WD track and easy pedalling. At the 6km mark there was a gate. With a typed sign attached to it. The sign was in a plastic bag.

The sign read: TA 2020 HIGH CRASH AREA

In the next 5km, three 2020 TA riders have fallen and been taken out by helicopter with broken bones. This is a grade 4 track, slippery, rough, with big drop-offs. You will need to walk parts and look after each other. The road after forest is rideable.

From the summit to jetboat take time, more injured and a death in 2019. More drop-offs. The jetboat will wait, don't rush. Enjoy the ride/walk.

The Kennett Brothers Xx

'What is this?' spluttered Luigi, on his haunches, gripping the note. 'Did you know about this? What godforsaken place are you taking me to?'

'Relax,' I soothed. 'You need to learn to chill a bit.'

The Kaiwhakauka was definitely a grade 4 track, especially with the recent rain.

Wearing clip-in shoes was not ideal in this situation. I had bad history with being locked onto a mountain bike. Luigi had tramping style shoes so he was well set.

There were many small washouts and nasty little switchbacks just waiting to throw the unwary. I dismounted 32 times within the first 10km. I was counting with sadistic delight. More surprising was that I kept remounting.

Luigi was behind, walking with an unimpressed gait. Trying to maintain some dignity. Hey, he had the walking boots.

The Mosely DOC shelter appeared at the 12km mark. It was new looking and very homely. This was where we should have stayed. Would have saved $100 and it was in a pleasant valley.

The track opened up and became a 4WD track. At the top was a large pou. Luigi and I took pictures of each other beside it. There was a gate leading to a gravel road.

Luigi had been strangely melancholic this morning. He began showing some cheer on finding the gate – a way out. A couple of cyclists went by and he became positively ebullient.

'Weekend warriors,' said Luigi, noticing they had no baggage. He figured that this meant we must be near some form of civilisation.

The Kaiwhakauka track became the Mangapurua track at the 27km mark. It was great fun being on the Mangapurua. This was a well patronized track. It was undergoing repairs, especially under the sandstone cliff areas which were prone to slips. The cliffs were massive and towered menacingly above us.

'You would have to pay me serious danger money to work here,' I said.

There were many signs saying to walk your bikes through the slip areas. No one was obeying them and being the weekend, there were no workers about.

A mega ride and easily the best day yet, for me. Even Luigi begrudgingly actually admitted he was having a good time. The track was a great tourist drawcard and, as such, was well maintained. Even café cruisers could negotiate it. There were about a dozen suspension bridges to negotiate. Purpose built bridges for the trail. An unladen bike could be stood on its back wheel and rolled across. A bike with bags needed to be lifted over the abutments at either end of the bridge. This became a workout after half a dozen. But they were lovely bridges.

After WW1, the government, in all its wisdom, offered returned servicemen allotments in the Kaiwhakauka and Mangapurua valleys.

A story board had been erected near the top of the Mangapurua Track. It featured a topographical map in the middle, surrounded by photos of the returned servicemen. In 1917 the first settlers took up their allotments. They cleared bush and tried to make farmland. At its peak there were 46 farms in the valleys. Life was tough. The terrors of being a solider in WW1 possibly made life in these valleys seem idyllic. For a time.

They built a wooden swing bridge across the Mangapurua stream in 1919. This connected the farms to the Whanganui River and meant they had access to the goods the riverboats transported.

The settlers were counting on a more permanent bridge being built. This didn't happen until 1936 when a steel reinforced concrete bridge was built. However, by then most of the settlers had had a gutsful and were out of there. By 1944 they were all gone. And all penniless. What a have.

NZ wasn't the only country where servicemen were being conned. In Canada, soldiers returning from WW1 were given plots on The Great Clay Belt in Northern Canada – to farm. To quote one soldier: 'There are seven months of snow, two months of rain, and all the rest is black flies and mosquitoes.'

DOC now looked after the track and the Bridge to Nowhere.

We descended the track into the 'valley of abandoned dreams'. Deep in the valley we rounded a corner: The Bridge to Nowhere was suddenly there. A classic concrete bridge in the middle of, well, nowhere.

It was smaller than it looked in the pictures I had seen. Much like the Taj Mahal. Or Leaning Tower of Pisa. Not quite as impressive in the flesh.

The ride from Whakahoro had taken six hours. We managed to get on board an early jet boat at the Mangapurua Landing.

The bikes were passed along by human chain and hung on racks at the back of the boat. Light rain had begun falling. Like Fiordland, Whanganui was a giant sponge.

The trip down river took the best part of an hour and the driver had to resist the urge to put the big jet into a tailspin. It would have been fun but also carried the high risk of bicycles being jettisoned like frisbees.

It was a short cycle from the landing up to the encampment. An albino boxer dog came trotting towards us as we pedalled slowly up. Behind the dog followed a pig. The boxer kept anxiously looking over its shoulder to check the hog was following.

Odd. Very *Deliverance*. The albino. Only this albino wasn't playing a banjo like in the movie – and it was a boxer dog.

Whanganui River Adventures had a great setup at Pipiriki. There was a lounge, kitchen, bathroom and cabins.

'Ah, you must be DC and Luigi,' said the smiling woman behind the desk, a woman named Agatha. (She said a lot more, but I missed much of it as I went out to go and build a house. She was still talking when I came back in.) Okay, I didn't build a house – I'm speaking metaphorically.

But oh yes, Agatha did like to talk. She ran a good ship, though. That could not be denied.

The rain began in earnest at 4pm and only a sadist would willingly set up a tent in that when there were cabins available. The reality was that there was only one cabin available as the other was booked by two other TA riders, who were still to arrive.

I found myself conned into sharing it with Luigi, who swore he didn't snore. *Remember, it was Mike and Lou who were the snorers.* The cabin was fairly large and contained two sets of bunks. Between the cabin and the main lodge was an open grass space and I couldn't help noticing the large area where the grass had yellowed.

'What's that yellowed grass spot down there?' I enquired.

'Oh, that's where we had the marquee set up for the TA riders,' said Agatha, matter-of-factly. 'We had coffee and snacks in there – you know, that kind of thing.'

'Oh,' I mustered ,weakly. Weren't we TA riders? The bulk of the tour had gone through – true – but Luigi and I were still doing the TA. Perhaps there was something to this Lanterne Rouge thing after all.

We needed to know a combination number for the showers. That had been included in the briefing by Agatha but I was just putting the roof on the house at that point, so I missed it. Luigi, fortunately, was good with numbers.

The showers were built for dwarves. Or was that dwarfs, I pondered, trying to decide whether to bend at the knees to get under the spigot or to bend from the waist. The shower rose was on a flexible hose at waist height. However, if you gripped it in one hand that only left one hand to apply the soap. You needed another hand to wash with – or prehensile feet.

There was a sign on the door saying to conserve water – a sense of humour.

We were very muddy from the day's riding, as were our bikes. The accommodation also featured an area for bike washing, complete with brushes.

I hit a couch in the lounge. A hot chocolate and a packet of macaroons purchased from the lodge. Heaven. A sense of satisfaction from a hard day's riding cum scrambling.

Ollie and Kevin were the other TA riders staying in the adjacent cabin. Kevin was fit and looking to make up some k's the next day. He had some mechanical issues early in the tour and was wanting to make up time.

Ollie was on a much slower schedule. He had a very road orientated bike. More like one you would ride to school. It had narrow road tyres and full mudguards. One hell of a challenge when the going got muddy. The most catching feature of his steed was the large plastic box perched on a carrier on the back.

'The carrier broke,' said Ollie. 'I've got it cable tied and it seems to be alright. The load was too heavy.' He then went on to describe the load he initially had when he started his trip. He had built a plywood box to hold a violin and strapped that on top of the plastic box. Ollie couldn't play the violin, but he was wanting to learn while on the TA.

I couldn't help but admire his intrepidness. Ollie was struggling to do much in the way of k's each day.

Burger and chips were back on the diet as that was all that was cooking at the lodge.

Pipiriki to Whanganui

72km sealed roads, 5km cycle path

If snoring was an Olympic sport, Luigi would at the very least be on the podium. His snoring was incredibly precise and smooth. Slow, steady and rhythmical. Snoring symmetry if there was such a thing. So rhythmically pleasant it could nearly put you to sleep.

EXCEPT I BLOODY COULDN'T SLEEP. I had even taken an extra dose of sleeping pill but it was doing nothing. I had earplugs in so at least I could take comfort that if any angle grinders, skill saws or nail guns fired up I would be safe. I had plenty of time to contemplate all sorts of rubbish.

Luigi got up a couple of times in the night to pee. At least he only snored when he was asleep. I was looking for the positives. Eventually I gave up on any chance of sleep and plugged my earphones into my phone. I spent the night watching the Rake series: I had downloaded a couple of seasons onto my phone.

Daylight finally crept its fingers past the curtains and into the cabin. Luigi began fossicking in his bags like an overgrown mouse.

'How was your night?' I enquired politely, raising myself onto an elbow.

'Not bad,' said Luigi, briefly stopping his fossicking to consider. 'Bit busy, but think I got some sleep. And you?'

'No. No sleep. You were snoring,' I said, in a calm voice, still laying in my sleeping bag. There was no point in me getting up too early. I could be packed in 10 minutes. Luigi needed more like an hour.

'Ummm, are you sure?' asked Luigi.

'Doing the maths, I think there's a fair chance it was you. I was awake so that only left you.'

'It could have been an animal that got in here in the night.'

'Funny that it made its escape at exactly the same time you woke up. I think you conned me, told me you weren't a snorer. That it was Mike and Lou. You knew all along.'

'It could be a first,' said Luigi, rubbing his chin in contemplation. 'It may not have happened before.'

'I think you set me up,' I rebuffed, still using a calm voice.

'Look,' said Luigi, urgency building in his voice. 'Please, whatever you do. Don't mention this to my wife.'

Clearly, Luigi was in some kind of denial. I noticed how he wouldn't even use the word, *snore*. But I tried not to get riled over it; I was trying to look on the humorous side. It certainly wasn't the first time and wouldn't be the last on this tour that my sleep would be disturbed. I had to become zen-like and go with the flow.

Luigi was a fluffer when it came to packing. Who knew what he was doing head down in his bike bags? But there was a lot of shuffling. Then a long sigh. Then more shuffling. Possibly an, 'Aha.' More shuffling. Pursing of the lips and … more shuffling.

By contrast, I had it down to a T and knew exactly which pannier things went in and in which order. To be honest, I didn't really have much. A spare pair of shorts, socks, two shirts, a windbreaker and compact puffer jacket went into one pannier, along with my toiletries and medical supplies. The stove, dehydrated meals, teabags, honey, rolled oats, bananas, OSM bars in the other. The front roll bag contained two lightweight sleeping bags, an air mattress, a tent and a proper raincoat, which would be gold if the weather ever turned real nasty.

On the outside of one pannier I had bungeed the spare tyre and on the other I had my jandals. The bottle of meths went into a bottle cage on the frame. Electrolyte into another. My stainless-steel thermal cup into a cage in front of the bottom bracket. Three litres of water into the drainpipe which was hose-clamped to the front tube.

After a full cooked breakfast, we hit the road. Kevin was long gone and Ollie was delaying his leaving to rest up a little more – to work on his spiccato.

The heavy overnight rain had ceased, leaving wet roads and streaming hills – pretty typical for the Whanganui River valley. It was cold.

This was an interesting area in the young history of NZ. Jerusalem village was just 12km up the road from Pipiriki. In 1892 Suzanne Aubert established the Sisters of Compassion congregation. It became a highly respected charitable nursing and religious order – and it was still operating.

It was where, in 1970, James K Baxter set up his controversial commune after converting to Catholicism. The poet and Māori culture activist was a polarising figure. His candle burnt brightly but briefly. Baxter died in 1972 and the commune was disbanded. He was buried there.

'Can you see that, in the distance?' asked Luigi, as we stopped at Jerusalem.

'See what?'

'That spire. Away in the distance.' He pointed.

'You mean, the church. Right in front of us?', I said. 'St Joseph's Church.'

I noticed Luigi was squinting intently. 'Is it? I don't have great eyesight. I had an operation in one eye that went wrong, so I don't see much out of that. And the other eye is average.'

Aha. That explained why Luigi always appeared to be cycling with blinkers on – looking straight ahead. Not turning his head to take in the sights. There were plenty of smells when you were pedalling – usually sights to go with them. *Was Luigi missing much of that?*

'I have a mark in my left eye, from the operation,' said Luigi. 'It's a small smear. Like lipstick left from a kiss. I call it Susie.' He laughed.

I was wondering how I had become a wingman. Especially now that there was some tension after the night's snoring performance. I liked to ride alone, a bit of company in the evening could be a good thing, but

I mostly liked to do my own thing, in my own time. To be able to stop for a leak on the side of the road without being asked what happened – and why the stop.

At Jerusalem Luigi urged me to film him reciting the Baxter poem: 'On the Death of Her Body.'

I got my phone/camera position and Luigi stationed himself by a ramshackle bus shelter and dramatically lifted an arm towards the church.

'It is a thought breaking the granite heart
Time has given me, that my one treasure
Your limbs, those passion-vines, your bamboo body

Should age and slacken, rot
Some day in a ghastly clay-stopped hole.
They led me to the mountains beyond pleasure

Where each is not gross body or blank soul
But a strong harp the wind of genesis
Makes music in. Such resonant music

That I was Adam…'

'Bravo!' I shouted. It was an animated performance that greatly appealed to my ken. It also helped me in appreciating the different angle Luigi brought to the tour. He wasn't your Joe Average.

'What? – I haven't finished!' shouted Luigi.

'What do you mean? That was fantastic!' I enthused.

'It wasn't the end,' called Luigi, huffily. 'There's four more lines.'

'But you stopped,' I rebutted.

'No. I paused for effect.'

'Well, I didn't know that. I thought it was the end,' I said. 'I didn't want to waste tape in my phone.'

'What bastard tape!' yowled Luigi. 'It's a bloody phone – not a reel to reel.'

Luigi walked his bike slowly back to me.

'Okay, true' I agreed. 'I will turn it on again. You can finish the poem.'

'You can't just start again somewhere in the poem. It has to be done in order.'

'Okay, sorry about that,' I said. Then I brightened, 'Shall we do it again?'

'No,' mumbled Luigi. 'The moment's gone.'

Oh well. Good bloody job – one back for me. The feckin snorer.

Rocks were spread across the road at many of the corners – the result of the heavy overnight rain. It was amazing that no rocks fell while we were cycling; it was not really a place to hang about – we needed to keep moving. The sandstone cliffs above the road were immense. Buff grey and brown projections. The whole river valley looked like it could come down with one good shake. NZ wasn't called the Shaky Isles for nothing.

A cafe/gallery was open at Matahiwi. It was in a delightful old whitewashed timber building. There were also cabins out the back. Matahiwi was a small village of slightly rundown houses. A farm dog was sitting outside the café as they rode in. Beside it sat a pig.

Odd, very odd. There's got to be something in the water in this area. Or the dogs' bowls at least.

A lovely elderly Māori lady ran the store. She said it was open for TA riders and she would close it up that very day, as we were the last passing through.

The Lanterne Rouge.

The baking was fabulous. We ordered milkshakes and I bought a huge cheese scone for later in the day. It may have been an isolated hamlet in the back of beyond, but the woman knew how to charge city prices. She was as sharp as she was sweet. Still, any place open was worth it.

It was a hard climb out of the valley. That muddy river wouldn't let us go – it felt like its claws were into us – trying to drag us back down. Light showers fell as we climbed. Eventually we crested the Gentle Annie hill. There was a lookout beside the road. I put on a brew to celebrate the climb.

A cool Southerly blew so we didn't hang around for long. Then it was a straightforward 15km into a headwind to the city of Whanganui.

The Whanganui River was there again to greet us as we pulled into the information centre. Muddy waters. At Whanganui it became a broad expanse of slow moving water. Logs and debris lined the banks.

After three days in the bowels of the Whanganui River valleys, Luigi and I felt like missionaries who had come out of the depths of the jungle and back to civilisation. (Apocalypse Now: We had eluded the Vietcong, killed Kurtz, and paddled our waka to freedom.)

Accommodation that night was at the College House Backpackers. Luigi got the room with the double bed. I got the room with the single but it did have an en-suite. The en-suite was a little make up in lieu of being forced to share a cabin the night before with the snorer. The backpackers was basic and suited us exactly – we were able to wheel our bikes into our rooms; no pretentiousness in this pad.

The Rutland Arms Inn served old fashioned meals. The weary travellers tried to muster enthusiasm to eat but tiredness had exhausted our hunger. We ended up eating for fuel despite the food being great.

Luigi went for some red wine. He raised a tired toast. 'A quote: "Most days I juggle everything quite well, on the other days there's always red wine."'

I raised my ginger ale to endorse. It took all my effort to eat – my eyes wanted to close. I'd fallen asleep once before while eating and skewered my nose with the fork.

Whanganui to Rangiwahia

70km seal, 32km gravel

I awoke refreshed – well, as refreshed as I ever was when taking a sleeping pill each night. I could never fathom why sleeping pills made you so sleepy and groggy the next day. They did help you sleep, more like knock you out, but surely you should feel awake the next day. You've had a night's sleep but you can't seem to escape the sleeps tendrils. *Sleep won't let me go, it still wants a piece of me.*

I found that it took the first couple of hours cycling to rid myself of the grogginess. The first hour, especially, was always tough. I tried not to think too much. In fact, I tried not to think at all.

I considered: Women had a problem with this concept. They couldn't fathom that a man had the ability not to think. The cerebral mechanism could stall out in neutral for some time. (Was it Einstein who said…No wait, it was Seinfeld. 'Woman always want to know what you're thinking. "Go on, tell me what you're thinking." 'We're thinking nothing.')

First port of call was the supermarket as it opened at 7am. I needed to resupply. Apples, bananas, OSM bars, teabags. Bags of milk powder and rolled oats. It was an odd look, rolling a shopping trolly to a bicycle to unload. A grown man packing food onto a bicycle; unusual character. Where's his ute?

It was usually the 'n'er do wells' who were intrigued and asked questions about what I was doing and where I was going. Your average shopper would smile grimly and subtly try to avoid any contact.

I enjoyed the rare experience of feeling like an outsider – seeing how the other half lived.

The problem with my shopping items was that I only needed a portion of the powder and oats – not even half of the amount. Otherwise, it was too much weight. I wanted to give away the rest, if possible. But how? Picture a man in camo pants, stained shirt, a skull cap under his helmet, with a bike featuring all sorts of crap tied to it – and a flag. He's in the carpark of Countdown with a bag of white powder, trying to make eye contact with people: Want some? Want it? The people keep moving. Not a good look.

Then there was the carpark cream administration. Being caught with one's hands down one's pants was never going to be an easy explanation. How do you tell someone you're just applying butt cream? *How do you even go about beginning that conversation?*

Second port of call was Velo Ronny's Bicycle Store. TA riders often got immediate attention when they approached a bike shop. They liked to think it was because they were special and on a great quest. Somehow it was vital for the shop mechanic to give them priority, get them serviced and on their way to the grail. The awful truth was that the bike shop owner didn't want them loitering around in the store – usually smelly, unkempt and dishevelled, the TA rider wasn't a great attractant for mum and the kids who were looking to purchase a bike.

Velo's mechanic helped me clean and degrease my bike in the wash bay. Who knew what diseases it had picked up in the Heart of Darkness? We had to remove the flagpole as it hit the ceiling in the workshop area. It was the first flagpole the mechanic had seen on a TA bike. I was proud of that.

It was up on the work stand. New rear brake pads and a new rear tyre and tube.

Luigi took his bike to a different shop, one that stocked Surly brake pads – his front pads were shot.

I popped round the corner to the Mud Duck's Café for breakfast while the work was going on. An omelette and more tea vicar. Luigi joined me.

'Did you know that I've spent a few Christmas nights in this town?' I said.

'Why would you do that?' asked Luigi, eagerly scrolling through the menu. He glanced up. 'And you didn't spend Christmas day?'

'No. I would fly in on Christmas afternoon.' I paused to remember. 'Then, Air NZ cut off the service to Whanganui. I had to fly into Palmy and drive the truck down from there. I sometimes used to park it at a lockup in Palmy between races. I raced motorbikes a bunch of times through this town.'

Indeed, I had raced several times at the 'Cemetery Circuit', held every Boxing Day in the heart of Whanganui. The street circuit was so named because of the cemetery in the centre of it. The Whanganui track had a lot more in the way of curious obstacles than Paeroa, but it wasn't as fast. In fact, on my GSXR1100, I would ride the whole circuit in second gear. I had at other times run an Aprilia RSV1000R and an F3 Kawa/ Honda – 'Frankenstein'.

The start line was halfway down the front straight.

I was never good off the line; I took a certain perverse pride in being a poor starter. The gist of it was that I liked to chase – enjoyed a target. I was hopeless leading and would fluff his lines. From the gun, the first corner (the track went clockwise) was usually mayhem with more bikes than room. I loved the Whanganui start – elbows out, lots of back brake and make like it's a motocross start: engage second gear and dive in. Air fences on the outside, orange plastic barriers and deer fencing on the inside. It was a frantic squirt of full throttle to turn two, still clockwise. Stay inside as you could easily get picked off here – no sweeping line at turn two. A manhole cover was placed a metre in from the kerb. It was better to go inside it but this meant you hit a sharp depression with a jolt – a brief moment of painful empathy for the machine. Then it was full noise down the back straight, with plenty of wheelies as the bike tried to hook traction. The next move was a right left chicane over a railway line. You hit the line on an angle (careful if it was wet). There was a chance for an overtake here but you needed to be sure you could get it done – it was the scene of many crashes and a popular viewing spot. The chicane set you up and gave you flow for the next section. A shipping container was mounted above the next corner as a walkway over the track. The road had a ridge in it here. The best approach was from hard left after the chicane, apex earlyish to the right, make sure to get inside the manhole cover, then pull it hard left, hit the throttle and turn it over the ridge on the back wheel – bum rising just off the seat and using the footpegs to help steer.

This was where the road ran dead centre through the cemetery – the ghosts must have got a hell of a shock. This was also the spot you knew you were riding a living creature. The bike would headshake and fight. I would soothe: *'Whoa, girl. Whoa, boy. Sit, you bastard.'* Whatever worked. I wasn't one of those Nancies who put a gender on his bike. It was a machine to do a job for me. I also didn't like a bike to be too flash. I needed to be able to crash it without feeling bad about scratching the new paint job. Sure, I liked it to have a certain look – my bikes were always distinctive – but a few cable ties and a bit of duct tape weren't out of place. If it was too flash I wouldn't push it as hard. *Function over form, lad.*

'And this was all legal,' I laughed.

'Isn't it dangerous?' asked Luigi. 'Stating the obvious.'

'Not as dangerous as getting between you and that bacon,' I replied, noting the fork to mouth speed with which Luigi was attacking his bacon and eggs.

'Just trying to catch up to you,' rasped Luigi, scrambled egg catching on his stubble. 'You got a head start on me.'

We were back at Velo Ronny's by 9am and did a quick scout of the shelves. I spotted some leggings that would come in handy as the weather cooled. They were more like stockings as they came individually. Luigi also bought some. Luigi in black stockings – I shuddered.

The mechanic was holding the tube that had been in my rear wheel.

'I replaced this. It's too large, it's the wrong size,' he said, authoritatively.

'Yes, I know,' I agreed. 'It's …' I was going to say that it belonged to the dolt I was riding with. But who was I to say such a thing, when *I* had been carrying a tube with the wrong sort of valve. Besides, it would have been unkind, and I was not an unkind person – except for the occasional thought. 'It's all we had,' I offered.

The new tyre was a Vittoria with a whitewall. Very smart.

Luigi considered my bike. He arranged his crinkles into a frown: 'You've cleaned your bike.' Luigi's bike was still filthy. He hadn't considered cleaning it.

'You can't break a Surly,' said Luigi, clearly a little miffed. 'You don't need to pamper a Surly. It's so strong, even with the punishment it's taken.'

With that, Luigi left the store and went to mount his mighty, but dirty, steed. I raised my eyebrows to the mechanic: 'I'm his wingman.'

The TA guide listed the Durie Hill lookout as the first target for the day. A 66-metre pedestrian tunnel took you from ground level to the doors of an elevator. Ring the bell and wait for the elevator doors to open. A custodian would take a small fee off you. The elevator then transported the visitor to the top of Durie Hill. A mammoth tower on the hill acted as a lookout. The elevator was 100 years old and the Southern Hemisphere's only public underground elevator.

The elevator was powered by a converted electric tram engine, and it was once lubricated with castor oil.

I had promoted it onto my bucket list for the TA.

Unfortunately, the elevator was under repair. Instead, we had to dig in and climb a steep hill to the tower. *Nasty way to start the day.*

From the lookout we picked up a glorious tailwind as we set sail into the interminable hills – more like hillocks. Pleasant enough up's and down's and it put some curiosity into the riding; it required a lot of gear changing. I had three chainrings on the front, 10 gears on the rear. It was change up, up and up on the descent, then all the way down, down and down for the climb – even a sniff of a hill demanded bottom gear from my carthorse.

Luigi had Godzilla turned on. I wasn't sure why but I dropped back to avoid getting a migraine from the flashing red monster. This had the usual effect of causing Luigi to stop and ask me what was wrong, and why I wasn't keeping up.

Oldfangled shearing sheds appeared, their yards full of ripeness – railings rubbed lanolin smooth. A top dressing plane could be heard working over the ridge. I was breathing it all in, enjoying the rural scene – classic NZ sheep country.

We were getting along just fine with the tailwind steady on our backs. March had just flicked over on the calendar. This was a great time of year to be doing the TA: cool mornings and more settled weather.

I spied a lone cyclist up the road, moving in the same direction. We were gaining steadily on him.

'Hey,' yelled Luigi, raising an arm and pointing ahead. 'There's a cyclist ahead.'

I shook my head. *I'm following a blind man.* If Luigi was a Gazelle he would have been hunted down a long time ago. *I definitely must talk to his wife.*

The day before, Luigi had been telling me, that his retirement plan was to move to Italy in his later years – when he had dementia. He would employ a fulltime nurse. Luigi would stand on the balcony to his room, above the village square, and yell obscenities at the local villagers.

This was his retirement plan. It made me feel almost normal.

Luigi said he had no hobbies. He would also like the retirement home to take outings: to keep him entertained.

We soon caught up to the other cyclist. His name was Nigel. I remembered him from the Dargaville campground. Nigel had no bags on his bike – Luigi had yet to spot this. Nigel's wife was along for the trip. She took off each morning in their car and at a prearranged spot they would meet for lunch. Then she would move on and set up a base for the night. They had a large tent, so often she would erect that and put dinner on the cookstove. She was loving it.

Nigel, not so much. He greeted us happily. He too was at the rear of the tour and it was proving a battle. 'There's nothing in them,' said Nigel, pointing down to his thighs. 'They're useless on the hills.'

It was true. Nigel was walking nearly every hill. He wasn't a well looking man and it was to his credit that he was even attempting to cycle. His final destination was Wellington, his home. He said he would consider doing the South Island next year.

We made it to the Hunterville Café just as it was closing. Generously, the staff let us choose some food from the cabinet and said we could eat while they were cleaning up round us. Three guys, looking to be in their 70's, were just leaving the café. They were riding 'Adventure Bikes.' A BMW 650GS, KTM 890 and a 990, to be exact. Having a ball.

I raised a hand, 'You fellas are riding some nice bikes. Living the dream.'

'Taking the long way home,' said one of them.

'You don't stop riding because you get old,' said another. 'You get old because you stop riding.'

'Never pass a bathroom. Don't waste a hard-on. And never trust a fart,' said the third, squeezing my arm as he passed.

'You can see we've been practising,' joked the first.

'Growing old isn't for sissies,' I said, joining in the joke-fest. I really appreciated seeing older chaps out and about. I was astonished that *I* had recently turned 60. (There must have been a mix-up when they were filling out my birth certificate – a scruffy 5 could easily turn into a 6). Fifty felt appropriate. What was that saying: 'If you haven't grown up by the age of 50, you don't have to.' I had so much more to do in my life; I couldn't afford to be 60.

Another customer was also leaving. He was on a Surly and riding the TA in reverse; it took a certain type to do that: to swim against the tide. He was carrying some gear: full panniers, front and rear. You didn't see that very often. I wondered how he would match up in a freewheel comp – might have met my match.

'I like your setup,' he said, inspecting my bike, namely the drainpipe water system. 'Very inventive. How much does it hold?'

'Three litres,' I said, proudly. 'It also doubles as a rocket launcher.' One of my favourite lines.

'Well, that's handy.'

Most people, either didn't notice the drainpipe arrangement – how could you not? – or, chose to ignore it, as it was odd: wasn't the norm. So, then you had to confront the issue of the rider who created this bike – he was likely to be odd too.

This intrigued me. The mechanic in Velo Ronnie's had put the bike up on his works stand, right in front of his face. We even had to take the flag pole off to get it up; the only bike with a flag on the TA. Yet he hadn't once mentioned the drainpipe.

I lived in a cob house, one I had built. It had no straight lines – much along the line of thinking pursued by the Viennese/Northland artist, Friedensreich Hundertwasser. The ceiling was constructed in waves, the walls were 'organic' lime-washed cob and the floor was Italian tiles laid in a slightly irregular form. There was nothing about the house that was 'conventional'. Yet, most people, on entering my house, wouldn't say boo about it. I still wasn't sure what to make of this. (Perhaps a student could do a thesis – seeing, but not seeing).

Leaving Hunterville we had to do a short stretch on Highway 1. This included two bridges. It was a bit of a sprint as there was no shoulder. This was the riding that terrified me. Give me drop-offs on the side of a slippery, muddy track any day, but don't make me have to ride a stretch of open road with Kiwi drivers hurtling up from behind.

Shortly after that we turned onto Highway 54, which was more sedate and led to a slope called Vinegar Hill. Nigel must have slipped past us while we were lunching. He was down a side road, loading his bike onto the back of his wife's car. I pointed him out to Luigi, who was as usual oblivious to all going on about him.

'Hey!' screeched Luigi. 'Get back on that bike. Ride it, man!'

Nigel looked up and gave a wave.

'We can see you!' shouted Luigi. 'Get back on that bike!'

One of the so called 'rules' of the TA was that you did it unsupported. It was all a bit embarrassing having Luigi yelling at the poor old fella. I put the pedal down to go ahead – to get some distance from Luigi. I didn't condone him yelling down an old man who was giving it a fair crack. Hell, we were all old men.

'Hey! Hey!' I heard a yell. I swivelled to look back.

Luigi was some distance back and had stopped. He was madly waving. I swung around and pedalled back.

'Wrong way, we should have turned just back there,' said Luigi, as I pulled alongside. Navigation hadn't really come into play since I teamed up with Luigi. From Matamata there had been a group of us, so I just went with the flow. Besides, most of the riding had been on established bike trails. Taumaranui into the Whanganui River had been pretty straightforward. Getting out of Whanganui was easy as you just headed for the Durie Hill lookout.

Luigi's civilian job was doing the mapping and locating of power lines. It involved pinpoint navigation down to millimetres. Sending crews into deep bush to map out a power cable route. He had apps up the zoomba on his phone – which he had delightedly demonstrated to me. Topo, Mapquest, MapsMe, Scout GPS, Mapfactor. The list went on.

He had lights on his bike that could melt concrete. He had a helmet lamp that could be seen from Mars. These devices weren't powered by batteries. Oh no, they had USB ports, and in the evening Luigi would hook up a monster power pack he was carrying around. Proudly plug all his supertech babies into Big Momma charger.

Despite all of this state-of-the-art technology, Luigi had no navigation device to tell him where he should be going.

He had a wristwatch (probably given to him by a NASA pilot), which was solar powered. It would squawk when he made a wrong turn. However, and here's the big flaw, it wouldn't tell him which way was the right way to go. It only told him when he had made an error. *Think about that.*

It was like riding along with your maths teacher right behind you. Every time you made a wrong turn a piece of chalk would hit you in the back of the head. Imagine trying to make the correct turn at the Arc de Triomphe roundabout: there were 12 exits. It was one of the most useless pieces of kit that I had ever seen. I would have mashed it into a thousand pieces by now. Stomped the life out of it until it could squawk no longer.

'So, let me get this straight,' I said. 'You have all these apps. All these fancy gadgets. You do this for a job. Yet you have no way of knowing where we should be going?' I was flabbergasted. And slightly annoyed.

'I do have the map on my phone,' replied Luigi, stonily. 'But I don't have a mount for my phone so I have to keep it in my backpack.'

'So, it's in your backpack navigating the correct way, but you can't see it,' I said, barely containing myself.

'I realise this could be frustrating for you,' replied Luigi in somewhat of an understatement. 'But you see, Richard, my wingman, was the navigator. He had a Garmin GPS unit.'

'Should you not, perhaps, have borrowed that from him when you ditched him?'

'Yes, I probably should have. And I didn't ditch him. He became unwell. Exploded from the drugs.' Luigi considered for a moment. 'So now I have you. You are my wingman – to do the navigation.'

I had to concede that I could now do that: thanks to Mike downloading the Topo app and overlaying the GPS route, I now had a purple line to follow. And I did have a mount on my bars for it. But would Luigi trust me to do that?

Luigi was a man who appeared to want to be in control: to supervise. Lord knows, control was a loose term to use for Luigi. Luigi had discovered in Hunterville, much to my amusement, that he still had his room key from the Whanganui Backpackers. Also, that he had left his night-time hearing devices there. Devices that provided some sort of white noise to block out the screeching of bats and pterodactyls.

I switched the Topo app on and zoomed it in. The trail turned off the highway and onto gravel.

There had been murmurings about this stretch on Facebook. People saying the state of the gravel made it nearly unrideable. I was looking forward to finding out what all the fuss was about. It was stunning country and great to get off the beaten track.

The gravel proved to be nothing but ordinary gravel. It was probably the continuing hilly nature that put people off. You needed to be confident to enjoy the downhills and the uphills could be tricky if you didn't pick the line with grip. The key to riding gravel, I had learned motorcycling, was to use the next gear up – the biggest gear you could manage comfortably. That helped pull the bike forward, gave it forward momentum. If you tried pedalling too quickly you just ended up losing traction and spinning on the spot.

'The only thing worse than cycling down the hill on gravel,' complained Luigi. 'Is cycling up.'

Luigi didn't like to stand on the downhills, as I well knew. It was that cramp in his left calf – *Horse's arse*. Luigi was good on toiling up the long hills. He had a gear on the Surly that was ideal – I noted that Luigi never used his very bottom gear. Luigi explained that it was so low that in reality it was a reverse gear. If he used it, he would fall over.

In contrast, my bottom gear left me doing 5kph. I could walk my bike at 4kph.

We met a German girl coming the other way: also doing the TA in reverse. And also with full panniers front and rear. She was wearing light sandals, which appeared to me not suitable for rough gravel: you really needed more rigid footwear.

Luigi and the German began sharing their dislike of gravel. Nattering like two old fisherwomen. I stood idly, letting them get it out of their systems.

Several kilometres later we met more cyclists doing the reverse thing — a middle-aged couple who looked fit and able. They also had loaded panniers front and rear.

What is going on here? I wondered. I hadn't met any cyclists doing the TA in reverse, now I'd met four in one day. *Perhaps it's a better formula.* Perhaps it was more logical heading from the cold of the deep south, with the concept of warmer weather the further north you cycled.

Rangiwahia was the destination for the night. Rangiwahia Hall to be precise. Camping was allowed there although there were no facilities.

Fortune smiled on the brave adventurers. I had pulled into a driveway, just short of the hall, to wait for Luigi. There was a bucket beside the drive with a sign. 'Free apples for TA riders.' I was just helping myself when a van pulled up.

'Ahoy, welcome,' called the driver, through the open passenger window. 'Give me a minute.' I moved aside as the man then drove the van into the driveway. Luigi arrived a moment later.

'Perfect timing,' said the driver, hopping from the van. He was a tall, thin chap with flaming red dreadlocks. 'I'm Joe. Just got home. You must be some of the last of this year's intrepid TA riders.' Joe had a broad Scottish accent.

'Not sure about intrepid,' I said. 'But yes, we would be close to the last. I'm Duncan and this is Luigi.' We shook hands all round, ruffled up each other's hair and then sniffed arses. Joe's dog was in the mix, anyway. A large hound that looked to be mostly Huntaway.

'This is our place,' said Joe, waving his arm in the direction of a sizeable concrete building behind him. 'But you are welcome to stay next door if you want. There's a B and B. It's empty.'

'Oh, great,' I said. That sure beat setting up a tent. 'Is it yours?'

Just then a station wagon arrived in a flurry of dust. A woman, in gay colours complete with a swirly skirt, sprang lightly from it and joyously embraced Joe. The embrace included a full blooded and lingering kiss.

The women are indeed hot-blooded about these parts, I thought. It had been a while since a woman had approached me with this sort of sexual ferocity.

'Hi, I'm Lisa,' she beamed, approaching.

I straightened and covertly dusted myself. I licked my lips and pouted.

Lisa laughed. She shook Luigi and my hands – warmly though.

'I'm about to take them next door,' said Joe. 'To the B and B.'

'Oh, goodie,' enthused Lisa.

We dutifully wheeled our bikes behind Joe's vast strides.

'It's free,' said Joe. 'No one's using it.'

This didn't really explain the situation to me, but 'gifthorse' and 'mouth' were two words which came to mind.

The house was clearly old, sagging and in its death throes – the theme for many of the houses in back-country NZ. However, a bright coat of paint had been applied to the front of it in an attempt to put some life into the old boards. It was a villa and must have once been a grand farmhouse.

The house appeared abandoned. We put our bikes on the back porch and followed Joe. He was having a light wrestle with the doorknob but succeeded in gaining entry. It was as if the owners had just up and walked away. Or vanished suddenly. It was fully furnished. The dining table had all its chairs. The lounge had sofas. The kitchen had all its utensils, dishes, pots and pans.

'Surely we need to pay someone,' I offered, looking about.

'Och, no. It's free,' replied Joe. 'It's for travellers.'

Luigi looked sideways at me and found me looking sideways back.

'That's very generous,' I said. 'Sure beats camping.'

Joe showed us the bathroom and lounge. 'The bedrooms are down the hall.' He pointed. 'Help yourselves, your choice.'

The pantry was well stocked, especially with canned goods. Joe said, once again, to help ourselves. Whatever we wanted.

Luigi and I were by now becoming masters of the sideways glance. Still, it was getting dark and a whole house to ourselves. For free.

Joe left us, said he had things to prepare, before dark.

The house was clean. Rundown but the bathroom and kitchen were spic and span. No mouse droppings or streams of ants which you could expect in an old, abandoned house.

Luigi went into the bathroom to test its operation. The hot tap in the shower came away in his hand. He pushed it back on.

I went to open a kitchen window. The whole window fell out. I hurried outside and pushed it back into its frame.

The place was rickety but it would be fine for a night. *A whole house to ourselves – for free. Who can say that on the TA?*

Luigi had carried his bags into the first bedroom and was fluffing about in them, as was his wont.

I carried my panniers down the hall. There were two rooms left to choose from. One was huge with a slumped double bed in its middle. The other was more compact but it looked as if a poltergeist had only recently departed. Duvets, blankets and pillows were strewn about on the floor and on the beds. There were two beds: a double against the window and a single closer to the door. I chose the single and sat on it to unpack my few belongings.

The paintings on the wall featured a farm scene with a paddock being ploughed by a farmer with a team of oxen in one and a family portrait in the other, probably done just after the war years. A matriarch dominated the picture.

There was a large old wardrobe. On top of the wardrobe was a doll. A doll in the loosest sense of the word. It had a clockface for a head. Buttons for eyes. A long body made of stuffed pages of sheet music. Its right hand was a clothes peg and the left hand was mutilated. The feet were little bells – like jingle bells. The doll's companion was a small, white fox.

The doll was a little disturbing. I didn't linger there but I kept thinking of a friend in Wanaka, Simon, who also had a doll. It was a Chucky doll, complete with bloodied knife. Simon had the dodgy habit of taking it on outings without telling people it was about. He took it one time to the Phillip Island motorcycle track, in Australia. We were racing motorcycles at the Island Classic. A bunch of the boys were sharing a house and Chucky would appear on the kitchen bench, the dining table or in the lounge. He was even standing at the top of the stairs one morning and one of the fellas was so scared he wouldn't ascend until Simon had taken him away.

Chucky went to the track with us each day and, while many thought it was fun to have him about, most were a little distraught. Chucky ended up wreaking havoc on the Kiwi team. Simon's bike blew up in the first lap of the first race. Two boys in the team ended up in hospital with serious injuries. Another half a dozen bikes terminated themselves leaving the Kiwis struggling to field a team.

You can keep your dolls, I reckoned.

The shower was brilliant, if you were careful with the tapware – a shower was always well appreciated at the end of a long day's cycling.

I had bought a slice of lasagne and a Scotch egg from Countdown that morning. I burnt a fry pan immediately. The stovetop was either full on, or off. A microwave would have been ideal but there wasn't one. I should really have baked them in the oven – but a sudden irrational fear hit me. *Human body parts could have been baked in that oven.*

I burnt the outside of both the lasagne and the Scotch egg while leaving them stone cold on the inside. Hopeless.

Luigi constructed what he loosely called 'soup.' It was more like a slick of tomato paste with crackers floating in it.

We were tired, so knackered that we weren't even hungry anymore – food was purely fuel. It was late, and it had been a big day.

Barely any talk was exchanged and it was to bed straight after eating. Neither of us wanted to give voice to any feeling of foreboding. (To admit we could be scared of the dark. Or the bogeyman. Or that a warlock and a harpy could be our neighbours.)

I took a double dose of sleeping pills; it could be good to be unconscious if things began moving about the house.

Rangiwahia to Pahiatua

61km seal, 49km gravel, 17km cycle path

We were up early myopically bumping around sorting our gear. Sunrise was still 30 minutes away. I dragged my bits and pieces into the kitchen to join Luigi.

'We should get going,' he said, in a sombre voice. 'I hardly slept. Couldn't lock my door.'

'I took double pills,' I admitted, somewhat groggily. 'My door wouldn't even shut properly.'

'I spent the night waiting for someone to come,' gulped Luigi. 'Terrible apparitions. The inbred mutants down the valley, where no one goes.'

'Have you seen the doll in my room?' I asked.

Luigi went down to have a look. He hurried back. 'Sweet Mary, man. How could you sleep with that … *thing* in there?' He looked aghast at me.

'I figured it was better to know where it was,' I explained. 'I was going to shift it somewhere else. Like your room.' I snickered. 'But then I knew, in the middle of the night, I would hear the little bells. "Ching, ching, ching" as it marched down the hall towards me.'

'Right, let's get out of here,' snorted Luigi. 'Feck me.' He gathered his bags and hurried to the porch. Luigi demonstrated that he could indeed pack quickly if push came to shove.

We quietly rolled our bikes towards the gate. There was a tree nearby, growing out the top of a cage of bones.

Luigi paused. 'What the hell is that?' he spluttered.

'It's bones,' I said, calmy.

I was using my Tiny Buddha to convert Luigi's fear into a journey on tranquil seas for myself. (I didn't actually know I was doing this, but I did feel strangely serene watching Luigi implode.) 'I asked Joe yesterday about the bones. "Bovine," was all he said.'

'Good god, man,' stuttered Luigi. 'We need to put on some distance. Get away from this place.'

We shot our bikes through the gate in the hedge and mounted up. The day's light was just coming over the hills. Quickly, quietly we attempted to sneak past the neighbour's driveway.

'You boys are up early.' Joe was standing in the driveway, a cereal bowl in his hand. Waiting.

'Ah yes, well, early birds catch the worms,' I croaked. 'Too good a day to waste lying about.'

Joe smiled broadly. 'It is that. Great to be alive, eh.'

'Yes,' I squeaked. 'I mean, yes, it is. Thanks a lot mate for the accommodation. Very generous'.

Luigi was a bug-eyed mute. He stood beside me, his mouth open and his eyes wide.

Joe smiled and took a spoonful of his muesli. Or was it knuckles. Finger joints with milk. 'You boys have a great day.'

It took a few kilometres for Luigi to start breathing normally. For his heartrate to come down. 'Did all that really happen?' he tittered. Then, outright laughter. 'I can't believe it.'

'Me too,' I agreed. 'I will definitely have nightmares about that doll.'

'And the Quicklime,' added Luigi. 'Did you see that?'

'No.'

'At the other end of the porch. Bags of it stacked up. Mother of mercy.'

'Imagine staying there on your lonesome,' I said.

Luigi gulped. 'Please, no.'

It was another cracker of a morning. Cold and a very heavy dew sat about the land. Small rolling hills ran away into the distance, like giant donuts. Fog filled the hollows and magpies sounded from within.

I had my windbreaker on but the sweat soon began freezing on my body – I had to remove it. This made for cold riding but at least I wouldn't catch hypothermia. My polyester shirt began to dry – polyester wasn't proving ideal. I needed to think on this.

Luigi was still chuckling about the night in the ghost house as we rode into Apiti. The good people of Apiti had left a hall open for TA riders. Tea and coffee were set out in the kitchen. Little acts of kindness. The hot cups warmed our chilled hands. Apiti was another 'blink and you'll miss it' town of about 200 people – but it had a key – it was the gateway to the Ruahine Range.

Steam rose slowly on the road outside as the morning warmed. I navigated us out of Apiti using my new app powers. I noticed that Luigi, following behind, had stopped to remove his phone from his backpack – to check on my topographical work.

The next 35 km was all gravel. The gravel was in fine shape and on one steep downhill I hit 68 kph. However, the bike began weaving in an unnerving fashion. I knew from experience that a speed wobble could be ridden through, more acceleration could work. I also knew, from experience, that this could spit you off.

'Faster, Faster, until the thrill of speed overcomes the fear of death.'
— *HST*

Speed is your friend…and your enemy. I backed off slightly and the bike settled.

The hills were dotted with sheep for as far as the eye could see. It was fine sheep country. There were plenty of big yards and shearing sheds. Farmers were going about their work.

'Leave it, Ben,' commanded a farmer of his dog, as they worked a mob. I slowed my pedalling – I was hoping for a 'Get in behind' – however that was probably more a Footrot Flats thing. 'Leave it, Ben,' in a slow, low voice. Timeless. I chuckled to myself, thinking that one day it would all be a bit much for Ben and he would rebel. *'Screw you, mate. I'm having this one.'*

This was Toyota Hilux country. Nothing but. Every man, and his dog, drove one. Barry Crump would have been happy – and Scotty.

I waved to the driver of an approaching cattle truck. The man waved back, begrudgingly. A half-hearted lifting of half a hand.

The farmers didn't seem overjoyed to share their gravel roads with cyclists. They wouldn't wave willingly. They did stare but I couldn't work out whether this was through curiosity or whether the farmers just thought of us as, 'bloody nuisances.'

I was enjoying myself immensely on this stretch. Great country. Would be a shame to see it go into pines. Must be tempting though – easy money. It must be tough country to farm. Rugged, savage and a little hairy. *Like the women.*

There was plenty of time to think on the TA. Those first couple of hours each morning were tedious. Trying to wear off the effects of the sleeping pills. Grogginess, however, was my friend this morning after the night spent in the ghost house. The nightmares were being held at bay.

The Waterford Café was closed, of course. We carried on and I did the donkeywork into a mild headwind as we approached Ashhurst. Luigi tucked in behind getting a good draft. The café at Ashhurst was just about to close. The woman let us choose something from the cabinet while she created milkshakes. We made the café only by the hair of our chinny-chin-chins. A lucky break on the café front.

There was a new swing bridge at Ashhurst, specifically built for cyclists and it also marked the beginning of a cycle trail into Palmerston North. Navigation wasn't needed here, so Luigi took over the lead role. His taking over also coincided with us picking up a tailwind. It made him look like Lance Armstrong as he powered away.

'Anything you want in Palmy?' I asked, pedalling my cycle alongside Luigi's.

'Nope' replied Luigi, smoothly into his work. 'You?'

'No.'

'What's the best thing about Palmy?' called Luigi.

'What?'

'Leaving it.'

'Ha, bad experiences?' I asked.

'Cold. Windy. Hole,' replied Luigi.

We managed to bypass most of Palmerston North to get ourselves onto the Pahiatua Saddle. It began calmly enough with a gentle incline. It even included a shoulder to lure the unwary cyclist into a false sense of wellbeing. However, about 10 kilometres in and it suddenly pitched upwards to climb 300 metres within 5km – and the shoulder disappeared. It was a popular route, in reality the only route, as the Manawatu Gorge Road had been closed for some time due to slips. There was no avoiding the close quarter encounters with cars, fully laden trucks and trailers.

Luigi got into his groove and rode slowly to the top. Meanwhile I was off my bike and walking for most of the 5km. I had to admit that nearly all of the drivers did their best to give me a little room. At least the steep and winding nature of the saddle road slowed the traffic.

Luigi was waiting at the top. 'That wasn't fun,' he declared.

'A day in the trenches,' I agreed.

'Have you seen any TA riders in the past few days?' he asked, leaning on his bars.

I considered. 'Yes, we saw those four riders a couple of days ago.'

'All going north,' said Luigi. 'Have you seen any going south?'

I thought again. 'No.'

'I am afraid, old chook, we are now the detritus of the tour.' Luigi laughed. 'Left over broken little bits of skin. Even the Lanterne Rouge may have passed us by.'

I powered down the other side of the Pahiatua Saddle on the tail of a white people mover. I was cutting loose as I could corner so much faster than most cars. The driver kept glancing in his wing mirror – the cyclist kept filling it. I was having such a good time that I flew past the turnoff and didn't realise for a few kilometres. I didn't check my Topo app until the road flattened out. *Whoops.* If I had a Luigi watch it would now be going berserk. Squawking like a manic parrot.

I pulled a U-turn and climbed the few kilometres back to the Ballance Valley Road turnoff. I then turned onto a gravel road, Tararua Rd. Luigi must be long gone by now, I thought. He would be dazed and confused not knowing what had happened to me. Why I hadn't waited. Luigi hated it when I didn't wait.

Ah, let him suffer. Will do him good.

A couple of corners later and there was Luigi, waiting at the side of the road. He had his phone out and was scanning it for clues.

'Thought you'd lost me,' he said, looking at me expectantly. 'Thought you might have taken off.'

'No, not me,' I laughed. 'Just got a bit carried away with the downhill. Shot right past the turnoff.'

'Yeah, I figured that might have happened. I knew you wouldn't have left me.'

Mmmn, I considered thoughtfully. *But I could have.*

We rode into Pahiatua.

'It looks like they're digging the town up to remove it,' I said, noting large trenches dug into the footpaths of Pahiatua.

Pahiatua had the feel of a worn-out town. It needed a good shake, like an old rug. Like an old golden retriever that needed a good brushing. Many of the shops were empty. Once a busy stop on the main trunk line, Pahiatua was now gasping for breath

'Fibre,' said Luigi, knowledgeably. 'They're putting in new fibre. High speed internet. That's why they're digging up the paths.'

Perhaps there was life in the old dog, Pahiatua.

Taito, my mate, had recommended the Club Hotel. He wouldn't say why but just that it would be worth it. I had booked but needn't have bothered; we were the only customers. Paint was faded and peeling on the Club Hotel. The windows had chipped putty and cracked glazing. There didn't appear to be anyone about but eventually we found an open door down a side street and stumbled in.

Our cycle shoes clunked loudly along the varnished hardwood floor and onto a Scotch rug in front of a desk. Luigi and I gazed about in wonder at the foyer. Lacquered pillars rose to meet the lath and plaster ceiling. A chandelier shimmered above. Button back chairs sat either side of the entrance. The outside of the hotel may have been scruffy but inside it was a set of stately beauty. However, further observation showed that it was one of fading decadence; like the Rolling Stones.

Our rubbernecking was disturbed by a rustling. An older lady who looked to be Fijian was standing in front of us. She was also a trail angel. A Fijian angelic, mothering wonder. She had been sent to make our lives as pleasant as they could be, right at that moment. We were captivated – and a little befuddled. The angel took us under her wing and led us upstairs to the first level, her wings lightly brushing the doorframe. The mezzanine had a couple of tilt, tufted sofas sitting in repose. The floral wallpapered hallway was interrupted by double hung windows – lace glass curtains hanging at their sides. There were rooms galore off the corridor. We fellas could have our pick. The angel then took our dirty washing and said it would be ready for collecting in the morning.

The Club Hotel was established in 1888. Some would say it was now run down. Others would say its grandeur had slipped a little, like a tilted crown, but it was still regal. It probably wasn't the greatest investment. It had been up for sale in 2019 for $720,000. You would need impressive vision. (Perhaps a retirement home for geriatric, eccentric TA riders.)

The pub downstairs was your classic old kiwi bar. There were two patrons in overalls. Probably fibre cable installers, I guessed. Luigi ordered a large bottle of DB Draught. Classic. I had a ginger beer as I was still forsaking the grog. I did cast a longing glance at the beer though. It had been a long, hard day and a beer would be a fine thing. But no, stay the course, I told myself.

Pahiatua was indeed isolated in the modern world, as Luigi found out when he tried to call his wife on his cellphone. He was instructed by the barmaid to stand under a certain doorway – that was where the signal was.

'She could have done this ride,' said Luigi, returning to his seat at the table.

'Who would, she, be?' I enquired.

'She would be my wife. She goes well. She's got an e-bike, but hardly uses any battery.'

I was amused that Luigi would talk about his wife as if she was an exquisite vintage car.

'That would make her a wingwoman,' I said. 'She couldn't be a wingman.'

'Yes. That's true,' chuckled Luigi. He poured another glass of DB Draught.

'Batgirl is the only winged woman I can think of,' I said.

'She's strong on the bike,' said Luigi. 'A good sportswoman. She did a ride with us to Horeke a couple of months ago. Made it all the way with two bars left on her battery.'

This caused me to hesitate. I went for a search through my fading memory banks.

'Did you do the Opua to Horeke ride?' I asked, a tiny electrode coming awake in the very back of my brain.

'Yes. It was our first proper training ride.'

I had done that ride. A couple of months ago. I had met two wannabe TA riders at the café at Kawakawa.

'Did I meet you at Kawakawa?' I asked.

'When?'

'When you were doing your Opua to Horeke ride.'

'It's possible,' said Luigi, frowning.

'You were with your mate, Richard.'

'Yes.'

'Richard had a chair with him,' I said, smiling as I remembered. 'It was a folding chair. He was carrying it on his bike. You might have had one too.'

'Yes,' agreed Luigi carefully, a captive note to his voice. He felt slightly like a fly in a spider's web.

I continued. 'Richard said, "I wouldn't be doing the TA without this chair." He could clearly see, *I* didn't have a chair.'

It had been a curious thing to say – and I remembered feeling quite inferior to the two gentleman I had met at Kawakawa. They had Surly bikes and all the bells and whistles; even folding chairs.

In contrast, my bike had a drainpipe hose clipped to it. A chopper flag at the back. A Homer Simpson figurine on the bars. A homemade frame bag. And stickers all over the bike from obscure sources: Roger's Yamaha. Pieter's Bier Bar. Motul Oil. Pirelli. Doc 2 Wheels. VR46. None of them anything to do with cycling.

'Yes. Well …' said Luigi, finding himself short of a reply.

'How many times have you used your chair?' I asked, smiling again.

'Well,' said Luigi, scrunching his brow in concentration. 'Not many.'

'Never, have you?!' I cried, in jubilation.

'Okay, that is true,' conceded Luigi. Pausing. 'But you don't take many breaks. We stop for a quick bite and then it's off again. I don't get a chance to use it.'

'Yeah, well it's slow going, mate. The only way we're going to do the miles is to keep pedalling.'

'That is true, too' agreed Luigi. 'If Richard had continued on the tour, we would have used our chairs a lot. He liked to stop and take a break. On the chair.'

We both pondered that.

'We may never have made it,' said Luigi, soberly.

We were knackered. Very tired boys. It was evening and all we once again wanted was to shower and hit the straw. The couple we had met cycling north, had told us to eat at the Post Office Hotel. Lamb shanks. And you got two, not one. Two lamb shanks, accompanied by roast vegetables. But we, weary travellers, didn't appreciate our dinner as much as we should have. The effort of lifting the fork to the mouth was considerable.

Then back to the comforts of a wirewove bed.

Pahiatua to Martinborough

111km seal, 16km gravel

The Club Hotel was a place where ghosts could abound. Swirling their lace and unfettered broderie up and down the corridors. But after the ghost house, it was tame for these two TA cyclists. Held no threat. We slept like kings.

Breakfast was laid on by the hotel. Toast, tea and Weet-Bix. Very Kiwi. We gathered our laundry from the angel. Neatly folded shirts and shorts. Luxury.

A light tailwind helped us into the day – although it went missing when we got out the back of the rolling sheep country. We were climbing for the first 40km, but only gradually. The metal road tracked the Mangaone River. It didn't have as many twists and turns but there were a couple of switchbacks where I could look back and chart Luigi's progress.

Rounding a bend, we found ourselves in Eketahuna. The cool thing about taking the road less travelled in NZ, was that you could pop out into civilisation at the most unexpected moment.

Eketahuna was home to a giant kiwi statue. I knew it as the home of Brian Lochore, a towering All Black captain – a man of both great stature and great character.

Eketahuna was also infamous in a book, published back in 2001. *Eketahuna: Stories from Small Town New Zealand*. A book that made author Peter Best few friends in Eketahuna. Perhaps more wicked was the Gordon McLauchlan book, *Passionless People*. He derided Eketahuna as an epicentre of NZ conformity. He described the town as a core where huddled 'smiling zombies' – lazy, smug and a bunch of moaners.

I took a photo of Luigi in front of the large kiwi. Luigi was ticking off the photo control points – a part of the TA. The kiwi was control point 13.

I was more interested in finding a cosy café as it had turned cold. There was a choice of cafes. There was a Bakehouse – a generic bakery in nearly every town in NZ. If you wanted good baking then choose a bakery staffed by older ladies – they knew how to bake. However, don't get your coffee from an older woman – unless you wanted instant. Get your coffee from someone aged 28 to 48. I chose the café with the most customers.

It was often tricky finding a place to stand the bicycle. A wall was ideal but usually not to be found. The bike needed to be stood within sight of the rider – there were plenty of light-fingered dudes in NZ. The trick to standing a bike was to wedge the back wheel against something. This usually provided a good anchor to stop it falling. Leaning the handlebar against something inevitably resulted in the bike sliding and falling to the ground.

Luigi had taken to waiting for me to lean my bike on something solid, he would then lean his bike against mine. I had let this go a couple of times.

'No,' I said, as Luigi maneuvered his bike closer to mine. I had selected a lamp post outside the café. There was a strong wind blowing and I didn't want Luigi's bike to compromise my insecure position.

'Can't I just balance it on yours?' said Luigi.

'No. With this wind, I don't want mine to fall down.'

Luigi began fumbling about, making a big deal of not being able to find an ideal perch. He tried this post, then that one. He considered leaning it against the café window. That was a no-no.

I left him to it and entered the café. I wasn't going to be drawn into Luigi's pathetic attempt to elicit sympathy. Luigi was a big boy now. If you couldn't park your own bike, you shouldn't be riding it.

They didn't have omelette on the menu but the nice young woman at the counter, after consulting with the kitchen, said they could make a three-egg omelette. I was happy. Combined with a milkshake it was the perfect protein boost. Luigi had a burger and chips. He was on a different food for fuel regime to me. Beer, burgers, baked beans, battered anything. A food group comprised of anything starting with B. *A B-tarian.*

Luigi, in exasperation, had eventually leaned his bike against a black Labrador. (A curious thing to do as the animal could flee at any moment – but) – fortunately, in this case it was a cast iron statue of a black lab.

Luigi cast worrying glances to his bike. The wind was beginning to howl outside. He gazed mournfully at me, much like a Labrador. I kept my eyes averted, taking in the artwork on the walls. I knew what Luigi was trying to do. *But it was not going to happen.*

The arrival of our meals coincided with the arrival of a herd of school children outside the window. They were being herded by a troupe of parents and teachers.

What with the wind growing to a gale, and now a melange of milling children, it was all a bit much for Luigi.

'Look, look!' he fretted. 'Those kids. Bloody kids will knock my bike over.'

Sure enough, they did.

(I fell to the floor, howling with laughter. Holding my sides so they wouldn't split open. Rolling over and over with joyful mirth.)

Okay, I imagined doing that. But how I wished I could do that.

'Whoops,' was all I could manage.

Luigi rushed out the door. He flung his arms about like he was trying to shoo a flock of pigeons. I could just picture him – bursting out of a vicarage vestibule, in a billowing cassock, arms flapping and clapping to vamoose a crowd of naughty children. Would make a great scene in some obscure movie.

The herd of children moved back slightly, as herds are prone to do. Safety in numbers. They didn't need to scatter as this man didn't appear much of a threat. Also, they didn't want to miss any action.

Luigi then moved to instructing one of the teachers. No doubt educating them on how to control children.

After moving his bike, Luigi re-entered the café and sullenly regained his seat.

'They are doing some sort of project where they need to note different pieces of art around Eketahuna. That bloody dog is one of them.'

'Good to see them out in the fresh air,' I said, somewhat lamely.

'Should brain the lot of them,' muttered Luigi. 'Especially the teachers. No control.'

'Mmmmn, yes,' I offered in sympathy.

'I think they've bent my derailleur.'

'I'm sure it will be alright,' I soothed.

The wind had turned into a howling Southerly by the time we'd finished eating.

'Let's get to Masterton,' I urged. 'I need to buy some warm gear. It's going to get colder the further south we go.'

I was still in charge of navigation. Luigi was still checking on me.

I was aware of it, and yes, it did irk me. The little things could annoy – especially on a trip such as this when one had plenty of time to ruminate. I was also still ruminating on the chance encounter I had with Luigi on the Opua to Horeke ride. My memory of it was returning.

I noticed that a few NZ Cycle Trail signs had either been placed incorrectly, the route had changed – or, some mischievous sod had turned them around. I was nearly caught out a couple of times but by zooming in the Topo map it was clear which way the trail went.

Luigi, however, was not going to follow me when clearly the signs pointed in a different direction. He would come to a stop, remove his phone from his backpack, and with great deliberation set about correcting the obvious error of my navigation. I waited patiently. Patience was a substance – like water. There was only so much of it and the pail could run dry. Inevitably Luigi would look up from doing his navigational diligence.

'I believe you're right.'

Well, yes, Luigi. The GPS map doesn't lie.

It was an easy run to Masterton. Rolling hills and mostly downhill. It was the first day of the America's Cup in Auckland. A beautiful zephyr blew them into Masterton – spinnakers up.

First port of call was a café, of course. Another omelette and milkshake for me and another burger for Luigi.

'Do you remember the Opua to Horeke ride?' I asked, as we seated ourselves at a bench by the window, in full view of our bikes. 'At the Horeke Hotel, I was sitting on the deck having a beer. I was the only one there.'

'Yes, that's right,' said Luigi. 'I thought it was odd. You didn't come over and join us for a beer. You sat down alone.'

I took a long pull on my milkshake. I smiled affectedly. 'No, *you* didn't come over and join *me* for a beer. I had finished the ride a couple of hours before you. I was already there – showered and dressed. You had just gotten in and went and sat at another table.'

I looked closely at Luigi. I wanted to see the cogs turning in the man's brain – to glimpse the reality cog.

'I don't remember it like that,' clucked Luigi, lightly shaking his head. 'Still, it was a while ago. I think you could be mistaken.'

Masterton appeared to be a tidy and well thought out sort of town. It was also a lot warmer than Eketahuna. Apparently, it received different weather patterns – didn't get so affected by the Tararua Ranges. It was part of the twin-set and pearls highway of NZ.

We finished our lunch and Luigi said he had looked at the phone map, that he would guide us to My Ride Masterton, a bike shop – to show he could navigate if push came to shove.

'Here it is,' announced Luigi, smugly, pulling up outside My Ride.

'Yes,' I replied. 'I spotted it the first time we rode past it.'

My Ride was only a few hundred metres from the cafe, as the crow flew, but I could have sworn we did 5km trying to find it. I also could have sworn that we went down some streets more than once in our quest.

'What do you mean? Nonsense,' said Luigi, as he went to lean his bike against mine.

'No,' I said.

Luigi followed me around the store, dutifully selecting the very same items. I gathered up some pink tassels to go on the end of my bars. I glanced sideways – Luigi paused, his hand hovering over the pink tassel bin. He blinked a few times in consideration, then passed on.

Neoprene gloves (proved sweaty), neoprene toe caps for the shoes (they quickly wore out with walking on gravel), a thermal skull cap. We also topped up on electrolyte tablets. I discreetly replaced the pink tassels.

I then got into a long chat, with the woman owner of the store, about Aaron Slight. 'Slightie' was a motorcycle legend throughout the world. A World Superbike rider, one of NZ's best. Masterton was his hometown and where he now resided.

Luigi was clearly less than impressed with this conversation and ready to move on. Outside the shop he bent down to his bike. 'I'm sure this derailleur isn't right. Those little bastards bent it.'

'I think it's supratentorial,' I said, wisely.

'Oh,' said Luigi, with concern. 'Is that bad?'

'No, you'll be fine.'

Masterton to Martinborough was still another 50km, making it another long day in the saddle. It was through yet more sheep country – there were some cows in a paddock to add a little contrast. I spied a three-legged goat munching away amongst them. Odd. The curious things you spotted along the way when you had time. And you had time. You could ruminate for hours, days even, on a three-legged goat amongst a herd of cows.

Pedalling was now like breathing. It didn't matter how fancy your bike was – whether it was a high-tech carbon fibre gravel bike, full suspension mountain bike, or a penny farthing – you still had to peddle it to get the job done. The TA Facebook forum was full of people asking for advice on how to travel light, or more efficiently:

- A hubometer would affect the speed/wattage output by 0.03 percent.
- The waggle of a tailbag drained 1.75 percent of your day's energy but was compensated for by being 13 grams lighter than a carrier.
- Cleated pedals were 2 grams heavier than plastic flat pedals but the 0.075 watts of power gained on the up-stroke made them worthwhile.
- A flexible solar pad could be carried on the rear luggage – it weighed 7 grams but it only produced 5 watts – on a sunny day.
- Lycra was the best material for wind resistance – flapping shorts made the ride 0.084 percent more tiring – but looked better.
- A single speed cycle with a 32-20 ratio would be dynamite on the flats but the hills would be near impossible – the end result would be slower than running gears.
- A 29'er gave you more roll over the potholes but was less tractable than a 26'er on the hills.
- 2.1 tyres on 650B wheels could be good but 45mm gravel tyres may be better in the North Island.
- Titanium bolts fitted throughout your bike will save you 2.5 grams in weight, but you run the risk of galvanic corrosion.
- Profile bars with 70mm risers are great on the South Island flats but disastrous on Big River.

You've just got to peddle, baby.

By late afternoon, my phone battery was flagging. Having to repeatedly pull up the Topo screen used a lot of battery. Luigi said he would loan me his powerpack to keep us on course. I could see that he really didn't want to; but it was a concession Luigi was willing to make in the interests of the team. Team Lanterne Rouge. There was no I in team.

I plugged my phone in and tucked the monster powerpack into my handlebar bag, securely covering and clipping it into the pod. It was as snug and protected as a Joey in its mother's pouch.

A few kilometres later Luigi drew abreast and indicated for me to stop.

'I think I'll take the powerpack back,' he said. 'I don't want it to get all dusty and damaged.'

'Do you think it will get dusty and damaged in there?' I asked, indicating the handlebar bag.

'No. Well, yes. It could.' Luigi frowned. 'Probably best if I look after it.'

I dutifully handed the pack back to Luigi. It was the little things.

It began raining an hour out from Martinborough. The going was easy but I was ready to stop. It was past 'butt hour'. Butt hour was mid-afternoon. No matter that I was now weeks into the TA, my constant companions – my sit bones, had still not signed a peace treaty with my Fizik saddle. And this, despite me continuing to wear two pairs of padded chamois shorts.

This was a 130km day and the day before had been 140km. On top of that I hadn't slept at all in the bunkroom at Pipiriki due to Luigi's snoring – the word that Luigi continued to refuse to say. Then there had been the night in the ghost house. I had gotten some sleep last night at the Club Hotel but it wasn't a stella night of sleep. What with trying to get comfortable on a centuries old sagging wire wove bed, my bum nearly hitting the floor when I rolled over. And the sound of flapping angel wings from the floor below.

It was time to up the pace, I wanted to get to Martinborough asap. I was very wet and now beginning to get cold.

Longbush Road became Hinakura Road. Vineyards began and soon thickened as we got into full-on wine country. We turned down Regent St. Suddenly we were there: Martinborough. You could tell it was Martinborough by all the Audis and BMWs.

We pulled up at the Martinborough Hotel and sat at an outside table – the only ones outside. It was cold and wet, like me.

I had been told that the Top 10 was a good stay and had nice cabins. However, Luigi had poo-poo'd that idea. He had been saying that he was going to treat himself in Martinborough. To go flash on the accommodation. He began noodling through the choices on his phone.

'Mmmmn, there's a lot to choose from,' he said. 'But they seem a little expensive.'

'No surprise there,' I replied. 'This is Martinborough. Top dollar.'

'There are some cheaper ones, but they're further out.'

'Okay, what have you got?' I needed to get moving. I didn't want to catch a cold. Even if it would be a flash cold that one caught in Martinborough. An upper-class cold that would require a better class of antibiotics to cure.

'Shall we get a drink, while we choose?' asked Luigi.

'No. I need to get out of these wet clothes, and soon.'

'Well, it looks like the cheapest might be $150 for a room,' he said, scrolling down the phone. 'And that's a few k's out of town.'

'Okay, let's go Top 10,' I replied. 'We've heard it's good.'

'Let's just see what's on offer there,' said Luigi, adopting the schoolteacher tone. 'I see they have cabins, and motel units. Those would be shared, of course.'

'Okay. Enough. Where is it? I'm off.' I got to my feet and grabbed my bike. 'We can sort it out when we get there. I am freezing here.'

The little things.

The Top 10 was superb. The showers were hot. I decided to take the next day off as a rest day. My knee had blown up after 270km in two days.

I was tired and obviously grumpy. I had been neglecting Homer. A day to chill would be nice. I texted Luigi to say that I was taking the next day out. Give my knee a chance to settle down.

I also texted that Luigi might want to push on and I would catch him down the road.

Martinborough

Day off

'Boom. Boom – Boom – Boom.'

I sprung bolt upright. *What the hell?* I looked madly about. I was in a cabin, my bike gear against a wall. Martinborough, that's right – it could be a little confusing some mornings.

'Boom. Boom – Boom – Boom.'

Okay, I rationalised. Loud, shooting-type noises at 7am. Why would that be necessary? Bird scaring cannons. *Unless it was the town square – the daily shooting of the peasants.*

Luigi was already gone – he had pushed on. He had left early, before I was out of bed. I wasn't getting up in a hurry. I had a kettle, tea, milk and honey. The bed was lovely. The cabin was great. I was in a cosy cocoon.

It was a day for doing basically nothing. I had a leisurely lunch. I read the local paper, *The Martinborough Star*. It was mostly filled with ads for real estate, by agents who looked like movie stars – and had names like Willy Cha Ching Harris, or Goldie ('just call me Gold') Dawnbreaker.

I went to a movie starring Denzel Washington. I was the only one in the theatre. Guess the title of the movie. The Little Things.

Part Three

Downhill, or Uphill – or Sometimes Both

Martinborough to Wellington

34km seal, 65km cycle paths

'In a little while from now, if I'm not feeling any less sour, I promise myself to treat myself – alone again, naturally.'

I stood naked in stockings. This was the leg warmers initiation. Trial and error dictated that they went on first – before the first of the two chamois shorts. You hitched the stockings up, way up high.

The day was cold. The first really cold one. There had been the cold and wet ones. But this was pure cold. Clear-sky cold.

My leg hairs were poking through the stockings, like Ena Sharples on a bad hair net day. I would need something to keep them from riding down. Like a garter belt – *was that what you called it?* I would need to shave my leg hairs.

My wife had also told me to go to the Glassons store in Wellington and buy some merino tops, to keep warm. The polyester wasn't cutting it in the cold. Glassons was a women's store. She reckoned I'd be about a size 16.

Women's clothing. Shaved legs. Stockings. I realised this was Transition Day. I was preparing for the South Island. Becoming Mainland Man.

I got my gear organised and mounted on the bike – I could do it blindfolded by now. I glanced across to the adjacent cabin to see if Luigi was ready; it felt a little strange. I was pretty good at chuckling to myself (and at myself) but I had to admit that if had been nice cycling with Luigi. We were different people on the same quest.

That was a beautiful part of doing the TA: it threw strangers together just because they could pedal a bike and found themselves in the same part of the country at the same time. Sport, in NZ, was like that. You could be a mechanic or a lawyer, but come the sound of the whistle, you were *teammates* charging down the field to get that ball. Afterwards you shared a beer and some war stories from the game. Come Monday and you put on your tie, or your overalls – different worlds.

I cycled alongside a stand of tall pines. There was no one about and the land was early morning still. A strange feeling began whelming through me – building as I pedalled. It was no road-to-Damascus experience – there was no lightning. Despite the chill morning, a warm fuzziness was spreading from my toes up through my body; engulfing me. If I had to name the warm glowing feeling, I would describe it as a Laphroaig moment.

It was a feeling I hadn't had for years. I was becoming a traveller again – not a tourist, a traveller. There was no longer that urge, 'must get there, must get there'. The destination wasn't important; it would happen, of course – but that was the end result. I was having something of an epiphany on this stretch. It was about the journey. The journey was what mattered. To focus on the destination was to weigh me down, like pinning a butterfly to a board. To take away my freedom. And that was the very essence of being a traveller – freedom.

It was a gentle 30km until the start of the Remutaka Cycle Trail.

'Paaarp, Paaarp, Paaarp,' a huge horn sounded.

I hunched down and hung on tight to the bars. A truck blasted past less than half a metre from me – easily close enough to reach out and touch. An 8-wheeler tip truck, towing a trailer fully loaded with a front-end loader. I held on grimly as the bike bucked and weaved – the wind rush nearly bowling me into the ditch.

I pathetically waved a fist and shouted some obscenities I reserved for these occasions. My warm fuzzy glow had been blown a couple of fields away.

There was no other traffic on the road. It was a long straight stretch. *Why would a driver put a cyclist's life in danger like that?*

I breathed deeply. I may have even made a soft 'om' – I was determined not to let some arsehole ruin my new zen state.

I wondered what a truckie would call that move. The, 'Old Brushback. Brushup. Brushoff.' Or just, 'I gave him the message.' 'Showed him who's boss.' 'Put the wind up him.'

I made it to the Remutaka Trail without further harassment; shaken not stirred. The grade was gentle but firm, like my doctor doing that unpleasant yearly medical check. It was a former rail trail so it couldn't be too steep: it climbed 350 metres within 10km.

By now I had legs that were strong. The rest of me still needed work but my legs were the business – they had been useless white wooden pegs for the first week – now they were tanned pistons.

It was a spectacular day and the Remutaka Trail was busy as a result. Mostly older couples and mostly on e-bikes. Fantastic.

The e-bike 'revolution' was in full force in NZ. Stats NZ had figures of 23,000 e-bikes being sold in 2017, 47,000 in 2018 and 65,000 in 2019. The Covid lockdown had blown those numbers out of the water – retailers had run out of e-bikes. E-bike sales had outdone the sales of new passenger cars.

I was overtaken by an older couple; old legs made young again on an e-bike. The woman made some light-hearted comments about me needing to up my game. I got them on the next downhill and returned the favour. Good fun.

I summited to find lunch was the order of the day. It was pleasant enough with a windbreaker on. Picnics were spread on the many tables and shelters. Cyclists all about.

Signage gave the history of the incline: The Remutaka Railway was built as part of an ambitious 1871 Government policy to construct a national railway network. Its aim was to link agricultural areas with major ports, like Wellington.

Mountain railways were a grand experiment in the 1870's. An English engineer, John Fell, had patented the first drive friction system – it involved a centre rail, elevated above the running rail, and gripped by a series of horizontal wheels. The specially designed 'Fell' engine was attached to a brake van and it would haul the wagons up. The innovative and bold system had worked in the European Alps and it would work in NZ.

However, as with all things, it became outdated after a few decades.

I was having a lovely time: no wonder the Remutaka Trail was listed as one of the 'greats' on the NZ Cycle Trail network.

'Spooky,' said the sign at the entrance to the summit tunnel. It was 500 metres long. I blundered my way through. Luigi's lights would have lit the tunnel up like The Blitz.

I serenely glided down the rest of the trail. I reached the bottom and was about to pass through the gate onto the seal.

'Wait, wait,' a voice called. A woman was jogging towards me; and making hard work of it. A middle-aged woman wearing a big smile. And clothes. The Wellington Naturist Club was still a couple of kilometres away in Te Marua.

'I'm Mary,' she gasped, gleefully.

Yes indeed, I thought. *You certainly are.*

'I'm a trail angel.'

Angels were surely out there, I reflected, as Mary got her breath back. The Club Hotel angel. The Dargaville angels.

Mary was responsible for the spread that had been left near Mauriceville – on some tables in a reserve with a sign for TA riders to help themselves. She was doing double duty and also providing refreshments at the base of the Remutakas.

'I thought I'd missed you,' she said. 'Your tracker stopped working further back. But here you are.' Mary beamed excitedly.

'Yes, here I am,' I agreed. 'My tracker – not so reliable. I've been kind of letting it go as it keeps eating batteries.' I felt a little guilty as people liked to follow the trail the TA'ers were leaving. But I also didn't really care as *I* knew where I was. Well, I did these days, thanks to the GPS download care of Mike.

'Luigi came through yesterday,' intoned Mary. 'I thought you were with him.'

'Yes, I was,' I agreed. 'I had a day off in Martinborough. To rest my knee.'

Mary smiled like a kindly aunt. 'He's missing you.'

'Oh. Right.' I wasn't sure what to say. I hadn't expected this. 'I'm sure I'll catch him up.'

I rode past the Naturist Club at Te Marua. A cold day like this: small peckers and large nipples. *No thanks.*

The ride down the Hutt River Trail was a blast, naturally following the river. The cycle trail was broad and easy. I met a couple of characters on bikes on the way. One fella flagged me down to basically give me a sermon. He began banging on about the means justifying the end. I tried to show some interest – there could be a nugget of gold if one remained open. However, I was downwind of the man and the alcohol fumes were suffocating.

I mumbled incoherently, waved my arms in big circles, and powered away: out-crazy the crazy. I wondered if passive drinking was a thing.

The next dude waved me down: 'Hey man. What is that?' He pointed at my drinking drainpipe. 'Is that some kind of engine?' He too wanted a deep and meaningful. No chance, I was on the move.

The cycle trail through Upper Hutt and Lower Hutt was wide and smooth. Touring NZ, I got to pass through towns with both European and Māori names. I ruminated on the imagination of some of the European names. Upper Hutt: I thought it was likely named for a building, perhaps an outhouse, or a stockade. The truth was just as exciting – Sir William Hutt was an English MP and a director of the NZ Company (formed in the late 1830s) and in part responsible for organising the settlement of Wellington and the Hutt Valley. Hence, Upper Hutt received his name. Lower Hutt didn't receive its naming until 1910. James Brown was known to be the first settler in Upper Hutt. *Riveting.*

I was born in Lower Hutt but had no memory of it, beside there being a large tree somewhere. I had left when I was five; it wasn't my choice.

The Topo line got a little blurry on the approach to Wellington. I reverted to the TA guide:

- ride along the stopbank for a few kilometres, ride under the Waione St road bridge, and turn sharp left, to cross on the footpath.
- you will pass Petone Wharf and ride through a carparking area, onto a path that leads to another carparking area.
- turn right for 5 m, through a gap in the flax, then left onto…
- La Cloche French bakery.

I was not good at following directions. I got to the Wellington CBD but not without some deviations.

People of all shapes and sizes were in a hurry. Wellington at 4pm on a Friday was in a buzz to get on with the weekend. Wellington had its own dress code – pretty much anything went.

Cuba St was crazy after the solitude of the back blocks. Buskers and performers were out looking to earn a buck. There was a guy blowing fire from his mouth, while balancing on a ladder, juggling live chainsaws and cooking a filet mignon.

A huge Cuban flag was imprinted on the side of a building. Cuba – an island brimming with soul-stirring music, vibrant art and villages cloaked in colonial charm. Cuba St, Wellington, was named after the NZ Company ship: *Cuba*, which arrived in the harbour in 1840.

As with nearly all areas of NZ, the history of settlement was controversial. Cuba St ran across land that was once next to Te Aro Pa and the gardens of Māori iwi who lived there.

I had booked an apartment on Cuba St for 70 bucks. I'd done it online and an address had then been texted to me. On arriving at the address, I found that there was a door but there was no way to open it without a swipe card. However, there was a handwritten note instructing to enter through the back of the Rebel Sports store in Cuba St. Curious. Like Narnia.

Indeed, there was a door at the back of Rebel's and I soon found the apartment reception. The helpful Indian chap on the desk gave me a swipe-card and a string of instructions on how to actually get to the apartment. He didn't hesitate at the sight of my loaded bike; bikes were welcome. I got lost immediately. I had to retrace to reception. The good man at reception then took me by the hand and led me up the lift, through a myriad of corridors, to a locked door. The swipe card opened this and I was into the apartment section.

My room was large. Large enough to swing a cat in – a tiger even. It had a double bed, a basin and a shower. No toilet. That was down the hall. And no windows.

I headed out to do my winter clothing shopping, before the stores closed. Glassons was close. There weren't any other men in the shop. *What a surprise.* The young shop assistant didn't startle when I enquired about a merino top. She gave me a couple to try on. The store was busy as it was a Friday evening. The first top fitted fine but it had a wide neck. The neckline hung out to my shoulders. It made me look like a large, hairy ballerina.

If I stepped outside that cubicle into the main part of Glassons, wearing that, I would empty the store. (I was disturbed by the apparition in the mirror. Imagine the public reaction!?)

I quickly removed the top and headed back to the racks for something more appropriate. A top that wouldn't require me changing my name to Natalia.

There were merino tops with polar necks. Perfect. The size 16 was okay but I went for a 14; a little more fitting.

After a quick and disappointing Mexican meal, I headed back through the maze to my apartment. There was a bunch of kids in the room next door – not five-year-olds, but teenagers. They had music playing. It was occasionally drowned by their boisterous shouting.

That's going to be a late one, I thought, resignedly. However, I was now in my new phase of chilled out traveller being, so it wasn't going to ruffle me. I would play it cool.

I put my bum against the wall and levered the bed across the room to the far wall. Away from the teenagers. Then it was time for a sleeping pill and earplugs.

The teenagers quietened down at 11pm. Probably went out to party. Then the nightclub below my apartment, the one in Cuba St that I was unaware existed, fired up for business.

'Oomph, oomph, oomph.' Fortunately, it was not an all-nighter and shut down at 3am. I practiced my *om, om, om* yoga calm breathing.

The neighbours in the next apartment, not the teenagers, but the ones on the other side of me – next to the wall where I now had the bed – had set their alarm for 4am. They rose and began their morning scrapings and rituals. It sounded to me like they were packing. Probably had a train or a plane to catch.

Wellington to Pelorus Bridge

Ferry 92km, 55km seal

I was up and away early. I was awake, so why not? I took the jerry can of petrol I had bought and poured a trail from my room down the halls and corridors to the lift. I then poured a trail into Cuba St and to the door of the nightclub below my apartment. A liberal dosing around its doorframe.

I then stood back and threw a match. I turned on Tom Waits and took in the music.

Tom Waits, 'Frank's Wild Years'

> Well Frank settled down in the Valley
> And he hung his wild years
> On a nail that he drove through
> His wife's forehead
> He sold used office furniture
> Out there on San Fernando Road
> And assumed a $30, 000 loan
> On a little two bedroom place
> His wife was a spent piece of used jet trash
> Made good bloody Marys
> Kept her mouth shut most of the time
> Had a little Chihuahua named Carlos
> That had some kind of skin disease
> And was totally blind
> They had a thoroughly modern kitchen
> Self-cleaning oven (the whole bit)

Frank drove a little sedan
They were so happy
One night Frank was on his way home
from work, stopped at the liquor store
Picked up a couple of Mickey's Big Mouths
Drank them in the car on his way
to the Shell station. He got a gallon of
Gas in a can, drove home, doused
everything in the house, torched it
Parked across the street laughing
Watching it burn, all Halloween
Orange and chimney red. Then
Frank put on a top forty station
Got on the Hollywood Freeway
Headed north
Never could stand that dog

If only that had happen – dreams are free, me old China.

I cycled the empty city streets to the Inter-islander terminal. A brilliant time to be cycling in the Wellington CBD. The early hours. You could ignore the Wrong Way signs and take any road you damn well pleased.

Covid was consuming the world, but NZ was doing its best to be a 'No Friend's Nigel' when it came to Corona viruses. NZ, Samoa, Tonga, Cook Islands (and many other Pacific Islands) had closed their borders. The plan was to hunker down and isolate – see what happened in the rest of the world and try to learn from it.

Tourism may have been the biggest economic earner internationally, but 'domestic tourism' was the name of the game during this time. Campervans were everywhere and tour buses were running up and down the country.

A couple of coachloads of elderly people arrived at the terminal. I wondered if that would be me one day. Good on them. They were still getting out and exploring even if it was in a controlled way that many of them may have found abhorrent in earlier years.

There were a few other touring cyclists at the Inter-islander terminal but they looked like weekenders to me. Their bikes didn't have the deep grime of a TA bike. Bicycles were given a privileged position on the ferry. There was a bike rack at the front of the bottom deck, beside the giant gangplank cum door. Bungee cords were available to strap them down. The Inter-islander was a well-prepared vessel.

There were the usual gaggle of Harley Davidsons being strapped down. Fastidious owners not wanting their precious Hogs to slide to the floor when the swell hit. (I should have saved a little of my dream sequence pyromaniac petrol for them).

I loved watching Harley people. The riders had come from the Hog Cloning Factory. Scuffed jeans, platform Harley boots, faded black Harley t shirt bulging over a Harley belt. A black jacket with Harley emblazoned on the back. Requisite goatie beard and wrap around shades.

'Chapless backs wearing backless chaps – knuckle draggers.' A friend of mine liked to say about them. *Hey, takes all sorts to make the world go round.*

The ferry was quiet. Nearly four million tourists visited NZ each year – but not this year. I found a table in the empty dining area. A power point jack was close by, perfect for charging my phone.

I glanced up from my electronic wizardry to observe a woman coming towards me. She was a large, unkempt woman wearing something close to a kaftan, and she was moving like a … 'ferry in a swell', was all I could think of. She bore down on me as if I was just a small dinghy in open ocean – *there's no stopping an aircraft carrier in a hurry.*

The fulsome woman plonked a tray of breakfast food down on the table right beside me. I was astounded. I swivelled my head – all of the tables were available. There was no one else in the dining area. If she had been an attractive woman, a moth irresistibly drawn to the flame, I would have been charmed. She was an abundant woman who clearly knew her way round a full English.

She could not realise that I was a misophoniac? *Why do these people seek me out,* I huffed, packing my few belongings and moving to another table.

I had been on the Cook Strait many times. I remembered a few rough sailings but they had been in the minority. One had been so rough that the kitchen was closed – even some of the crew had been throwing up. I wasn't a natural sailor. An oily, slow swell was the one that got me. Strangely enough, the rougher it got, the better I felt. (Now, *that* was one for the psychiatrist couch).

It was a great sailing, very smooth, and the ferry pitched us up at Picton just over three hours later. Cyclists were away first. I found myself standing beside a tall cyclist, with a basic older bike and no luggage. The man had only a backpack. He looked familiar. He looked like Jonathan Kennett – one of the three brothers famous for building cycling trails and networks throughout NZ. And the author of a myriad of books about them. The brothers also wrote the Tour Aotearoa Official Guide's.

But was it really Jonathan Kennett? I was 99% sure. It was usually the 1% that got me in trouble. I would play it cool.

'You doing the TA?' asked Jonathan.

'Yes,' I said, keeping it brief. *Damn. Jonathan would know I was, like, the last rider on this year's tour.* I wondered if Jonathan had given my bike the once over. With all its contraptions. Would he think that was cool? *Or was it ridden by a freak?*

'How's it going?' enquired Jonathan.

'Well, it was really hard at the start. I think I ate too many carbs. I had porridge on 90-Mile Beach and hit the wall. Then I had baked beans and potato salad on top of that. Which just made it worse. The carbs aren't good. Not during the day at least. They rob you of energy. All the body does is digest those carbs. The energy is all spent digesting the carbs. Then there's nothing left for the muscles. I've started drinking milkshakes. Protein. And eggs. Lots of eggs. The protein goes straight to the muscles. Milk. Lots of milk.'

I clamped a hand to my mouth. *What had I just done? Babbling like a mad chimp. Like a rabid dog assailing the god of the TA.* I looked aghast at Jonathan – who appeared surprised by the tirade. And slightly amused.

'I did the TA,' he said, pointing to a sticker on his bike. TA2016, it read. That was the inaugural TA.

'Ah, yes,' I spluttered. 'Good.'

Fortunately, the gigantic gangplank began lowering and the noise from it drowned out any chance of further conversation.

Must get away from here fast. Break for it asap. *What a dick I am.*

Jonathan waved as I mounted up and powered quickly away. A man of few words. *Bloody hell, he couldn't get one in with all my raving.*

I called at the famous Picton Village Bakery for a sandwich. The lady behind the counter said the pies were half-price and talked me into a Moroccan lamb. The pie, on top of a sandwich, made itself known as I climbed out of Picton – I had to take a moment and walk it off for a few km's. A mountain bike track was being built from Picton to Havelock. The first section was completed. It dipped and bounded through some lovely bush.

There was no one on the trail, which surprised me, this being a Saturday. I stopped at a fork in the track to take a pee. I'd become expert at being able to pee while staying aboard the bike. Straddle the frame and pee to the side. Okay, occasionally a sprinkle would hit my shoe, but hey, who cared. I peed off to the side, on the upside of the trail. The ground was rock hard. The pee began flowing back down onto the main part of the trail. The ground was so hard it couldn't soak in. It began to pool.

Just then an older couple of walkers rounded the corner. They hesitated: the woman looked down at the pee burbling across the trail. Horror flooded her face – she switched her alarmed gaze to me.

'Hi, lovely day for it,' I said brightly, looking away to the sky – anywhere but down.

The couple didn't reply. They paused briefly, scuttled sideways like crabs and took a wide berth. I watched them quicken their stride and scurry around the corner. I glanced back down to the little yellow pond I had made. There was no explaining that. The couple knew that. I knew that.

I would have wet myself laughing, but, as the French would say: 'Tant pis.' Oh well.

A strong tailwind arose. I got up to 30kph as I sped towards Havelock. The annual Oyster Festival was just winding down – people tanked on oysters and craft beer. I was a little concerned about being run down by a drunk driver on the road to Pelorus Bridge but most drivers gave me a wide berth. I was still chuckling about my toilet timing.

Pelorus Bridge campground was a DOC ground, $20 for a tent site. There were showers and a kitchen with gas cookers. No pots, pans or crockery – the usual story. And no power points – anywhere. *What's up with that DOC?* I needed to charge my phone.

I had bought mince and Uncle Ben's Rice. Sweet chilli rice this time. I had to cook it in my little Trangia pot, which took skill. The mince and rice volume nearly exceeded the volume of the small pot. I had to hold my tongue just so to make it work.

I was the only bloke in the kitchen. There were several women expertly working their camp cooking gear. I knew they had half an eye on me to see what I would concoct. Well, little did they know I was an expert in bland cuisine.

A couple of young women arrived by bike. I had seen them in the

Inter-islander departure lounge. They informed me that they were doing the South Island leg of the TA. This was their first day. They looked puffed but were having fun.

Camping cyclists had a designated area near the bathroom for their tents, which suited me. *Got to be careful where you pee.*

Pelorus Bridge to Wakefield

24km seal, 7km gravel, 29km cycle
trail, 12km 4WD track

It was a cold morning with a heavy dew. I had needed both of my sleeping bags in the night. It would have made more sense to have one thicker one rather than two thin ones. But I didn't. I hung the tent on the washing line to get rid of some moisture before packing it. Daybreak was getting later, as were my starts. 9am this morning after tea and porridge.

I began the day with my windbreaker over the merino. Once I began sweating I packed the windbreaker and just went Glassons on skin. It was a little cool but way better than sweating up a sauna inside the windbreaker – which would then turn to ice. This was the first real test of the Glassons merino top. And it passed with flying colours. However, once the merino top was wet, there was no drying the sucker in a hurry. I changed to my lightweight Nike Dry-Fit shirt when the day warmed up. I put the Glassons top on my handlebar bag to try to dry it in the wind.

The mist began lifting as I started the climb to the Maungatapu Saddle. The graph in the TA guide was horrific. It didn't seem possible anyone could get up something that steep – at least without ropes, crampons and yaks. It was an 800-metre climb within 8kms.

TA guide note: The Maungatapu Track is very hard for those on heavily laden touring bikes. The alternative route is Highway 6 via Rai Valley and the Whangamoas. It is a busy highway, with little or no shoulder in places.

'What do you reckon, Homer,' I said. 'Doable?'

I was feeling strong by now. The North Island had knocked me into shape. I had lost four kilos and my legs were strong. I was still on the Triazolam sleeping med at night: it gave me six hours of sleep. This meant, I was still a drongo for the first hour each day until I sweated the little pill out of my system.

It clearly said that the track would be 'very hard' for those on heavily laden touring bikes – but the alternative route looked appalling to me. 'Little or no shoulder in places'. The Maungatapu Saddle might be hell, but for me, avoiding the highways was vital. I knew that many on the TA would bypass the saddle. They would be missing out on the possibility of adventure – plus, it's part of the TA. It was a testing section. *If you want to take part in the Hop, Skip and Jump, you can't skip the skip.*

'And welcome back, little buddy,' I said, rubbing Homer's hair. All three of them.

Homer didn't reply.

'Hey, little fella,' I said, putting my face at eye level to Homer and tenderly squeezing his arm.

Homer was silent. I knitted my brow: when was the last time Homer had talked to me? *He must have said something in Wellington. Perhaps not. Martinborough, that would have been it. When Luigi left – I didn't have anyone else to talk to. Okay, when I nearly got flattened by the prick in the truck; he must have said something then. When was the last time we had spoken?*

I was pulling a blank. Dulp, I had screwed up. I had totally ignored Homer – for, crikey, maybe even more than a week.

'Um, buddy,' I attempted, getting down again to look Homer in the eye. Well, not exactly in the eye. Homer's eyes were casting off to one side. It was his normal, distracted, slightly scaredy-cat look.

'Come on, mate, I screwed up.' I was a little panicky. It was fine being alone again and able to do my own thing. To go where I wanted, when I wanted. I had also morphed back into being a traveller – *a beautiful thing*. But I was about to attempt the Maungatapu Saddle, for Pete's sake, and it would be very good to have a mate along.

'Look, I got involved on the trip and talking with Luigi, I know. I should have included you, but …' I wasn't quite sure how to explain this to Homer. *But you're not real.* (Homer sure thought he was real.) Luigi suspected I had a screw loose. If he had found me talking to the doll on my bars – *well, that would have been one way to escape the wingman role.*

I looked back down the way I had come. Giant electricity pylons filed away down the hills like silent Tripods. I was a long way from a town. I squatted once more and pressed my face close to Homer.

'I'm sorry,' I said.

'There,' said Homer. 'That's all it took.'

'Oh, buddy. You're back.' I laughed with relief.

'Oh. Buddy is it now?' replied Homer. 'Now that you've lost your bum-buddy you're back talking to me.'

'Yes, sorry about that, Homey,' I said. 'Why didn't you pipe up?'

'Hey pal, stop with the Homey. What could I say? You were playing second fiddle to Wing Commander Luigi. Where did that leave me?'

'Yeah, well the going's going to get tough now,' I said, drawing a deep breath. 'I will need you, Homey. I mean, Homer. Sir Homer.'

'Okay, smart alec,' said Homer, nearly smiling. 'Enough already. We've got this. Onwards and upwards. Well … upwards.'

DANGER, in bright red letters. Track Closed Please Keep Out. The sign was quite clear at the bottom of the Maungatapu Saddle. It also said: Open to Trampers, Mountain Bikes and Motorbikes.

How cool was that? Open to motorbikes.

It was a beautiful day, a fine one for walking. The track had some loose rock and was a little tricky in places. Very doable for an average mountain biker. I could have ridden more of it but I enjoyed walking these stretches. There was little difference in speed between walking and riding for me on the hills, so enjoy the spectacle, I figured. The view was magnificent. The track was basically a service track for the power pylons. I met a couple in a 4WD coming down the track. They were the owners of that block of land. They were laying wasp traps. Honey was a big earner for them, and the wasps were killing their bees.

A few kilometres from the top, I came across a sign, Murderers Rock. There was a display board giving all the gory details. The Burgess Gang held up and killed five travellers on that very spot in 1866. They were after money and gold having heard that a party was going to be on the Maungatapu Track and that they were carrying some serious loot. This did not come to pass but instead they robbed and killed those unfortunate to have been using the track at that time.

The Burgess Gang didn't seem to be overly proficient with their firearms, of which they had plenty. Their preferred method of killing appeared to be strangulation. Then stabbing. When they did use their guns, they either stabbed or strangled them as well. Just to be sure, to be sure.

The gang was caught. Three of the gang were strung up and the fourth – the one who ratted them out – got life imprisonment.

Well, I never. On this isolated track, on this very spot. Time to move on.

Not far up the track from Murderers Rock, I encountered a fit couple near jogging down the track towards me. They told me it was only another five minutes to the top. They also told me the downhill would be good with not much in the way of loose rocks (they were wrong on both counts).

It took me two hours to get to the saddle at 735 metres of elevation. 90% of the climb was spent pushing my bike. My average speed was somewhere around 3.5kph.

I didn't linger long at the top. I could see Nelson in the distance. The downhill was where the fun began; this was my heaven. There was actually more loose rock on the downhill than the up, however, that just upped the fun level. There was also a nasty rock garden section. *One man's terrorist is another man's freedom fighter.*

The best position was bum over the back wheel and touching the rear guard on some steep descents. A dropper seat and some suspension would have been nice.

What goes up must come down. The run into Nelson was quite magnificent. The Maitai Valley Road ran beside the Maitai River. It was a popular recreational area: swimming holes, a golf course, camping and even a dog exercise area – where I came from, we called that particular area 'outside'. The road and stream flowed all the way peacefully into Nelson.

A couple of attractive women approached me, while I was stopped, consulting the guide. (The guide said: *You will be approached by women of beauty when you enter Nelson. They are the Nelson Sirens. Don't succumb to their sweet lures.*)

The women laughed gaily and said they could spot a TA rider. *I bet you can*, I thought. They also offered me advice on where the best cafes were. (More likely, where their lair was. I wasn't about to lose myself at this stage of the tour. To be taken to my doom by these ravishing beauties.)

The women told me that a friend of theirs was also doing the TA. He had gone through Nelson the week before; a week quicker. *Oh.* My impressive ego spinnaker instantly deflated.

There were plenty of cycle lanes marked on the roads. Cycle friendly Nelson – probably the most cycle friendly town in NZ. It was very orderly after all the banging around on a rocky trail. I slowly piloted through the leafy and idyllic streets.

'Thought I'd lost you again, big buddy,' chuckled Homer.

'No, what,' I said. 'C'mon. What, those women? No, never.'

'You do have a vivid imagination, pal,' chuckled Homer. 'Just saying.'

Torpedo 7 was the place for supplies. I had lost my Mons top on the Remutaka Trail – it had been a gift from my family. I had misplaced my neck buff on the Maungatapu – a gift from my mate, Simon. The mouthpiece for my drainpipe drinking tube had disappeared. It was a time of loss.

I bought a couple of dehydrated meals, a mouthpiece and some more butt cream. I had gone through a massive tube of the stuff – *who would have thunk?*

I then got a little lost getting out of Nelson. My phone had gone flat. *Thanks DOC for having no power points at Pelorus Bridge campground. Very useful, not.* It was back to the official guide for help. There was a guide for the North Island and one for the South Island. Somehow, somewhere, I had spilt chocolate milk on the top of the South Island booklet. On the outside corner and the pages were now sticking together.

Nelson was no Auckland, but I kept missing the turn-offs. I could see the cycle track that I should be on, over yonder, it was just a matter of getting to it. I found myself sprinting the bike across a dual carriageway – fair game for Kiwi motorists. *Beware Molly Whuppie.*

I rode the sealed cycleway to Richmond – a town first settled by Europeans in 1842. It was remarkably unremarkable.

The Great Taste Trail really kicked into gear here (officially in Nelson, to be precise) and was perfect for the cruising brigade. Modelled on similar trails in Europe, it was mainly flat and passed through vineyard after vineyard. The Nelson region was known for having the most sunshine hours in NZ and if you were into fine food and drink, the GTT was the place to ride. (You could have a close encounter with a baguette, get plastered on a cab sav and wobble your way back home.)

I was feeling stonkered and decided to pull up at the historic Wakefield Hotel. I had read that there seemed to be some confusion as to when exactly the hotel was first established. The Wakefield Arms was established in 1853 (perhaps earlier) but it wasn't until Thomas N Trower applied for a bush licence in 1855 that its foundation was truly defined. *There was no buying a savvy blanc in those days.* 1868 was the big year for the Wakefield Arms. The Waimea South Steeplechase was held, and the hotel became the centre for the event.

The course was a three-miler and began on the Nelson side. It ran parallel with the road, crossed at the Hooper's Store and returned down the left side, passing through Mr Fowler's notorious paddock. The paddock was where things got gnarly as a deep drain awaited a tired horse and rider – falling in this meant the end of the race. There were 24 fences on the course; it was not for the faint-hearted.

I was delighted to learn that the long intervals between races were filled by the band – 'giving some gentlemen the opportunity to display certain steps which had not previously been introduced'.

The horses had magnificent names befitting a mount that would take on such a mighty event: Blundell's Deception, Baigent's Sultan, Knapp's Te Kooti, Paap's Blossom, Hatilow's Physic, Redwood's Bones, Monro's Rustic, Dillon's Quick Silver and Bryant's Minnie.

The fine lady of the hotel led me to a shed out the back where I could lock the bike for the night. She was proud of the sophisticated lock on the shed. It was a combination lock that was triggered by simply passing your palm over its face.

Fool proof. Except, I noticed, there was no catch for the locking bar and a small tug would pull the door open. *Oh well*. No denying it was fancy, though.

Breakfast was included in the price, so I had a late afternoon breakfast from the buffet. I then hung the wet tent on curtain rails and cupboard handles in my room. I boiled up a dehydrated meal, honey soy chicken, showered and hit the hay. Tomorrow, I was aiming for a 130km day.

Wakefield to Murchison

58km seal, 72 gravel

I broke my bike out of the storage shed – I didn't bother with the magic wave of the hand. There were saddles to be summitted this day. The advantage of staying in accommodation was that you didn't need to deal with a wet tent and all the kerfuffle of packing your sleeping bits. Probably saved an hour.

The Belgrove Tavern stood just 10km down the road. NZ once had watering holes strung throughout the country, like a pirate's necklace. In 1894 there were 1719 licenced premises serving a population of under one million.

The original Belgrove Hotel was built in 1856 but burnt down in 1930. The present building was built the same year. It was no easy feat making money in a country pub and the Belgrove had been sold in 2020 – another optimistic owner was now having a crack.

I remembered, back-a-wee-ways, that you were a legend if you could drink and then navigate your car home. I figured this was probably a leftover from the days when patrons would ride their horses to the pub. If, at the end of the session, they could somehow get back up on their long-suffering steed, the good animal would meander them home. I had recent recall of a woman in Greymouth still adopting that practice. I also recalled reading a newspaper report of a Dargaville man being arrested for DIC on the way home from the pub – of a ride-on lawnmower.

The 52-year-old man was seen by police at 9.30pm driving his ride-on through town. The cops asked him to get the mower off the road: they then discovered he was a disqualified driver and on giving him a breath test, found he recorded more than twice the legal limit.

The driver, Mr Gunn, was mystified by his arrest: 'I can accept it might have been a little dangerous, because I didn't have lights. But it wasn't DIC, because it wasn't a car.'

Mr Gunn was charged with careless driving, driving while disqualified, and driving with excess breath alcohol.

Nowadays you were a legend if you drove home sober – *what were you doing at the pub, eh, if you weren't drinking?* Unfortunately, drinking and driving had never truly gone out of fashion in NZ. I did think it was kind of cool though, it was the only Westernised country I knew of, where it was okay to drive while holding a beer – *so long as you were under the limit.*

I meandered along the GTT until my steed came upon a closed gate. My phone was now fully charged and the GPS map clearly showed that through the gate lay the correct trail. It was definitely a part of the GTT network (and TA), although it looked like private land. This trail led to Spooners Tunnel.

The information board at the mouth of the tunnel was very informative. Many thought it was a marvel that the builders of the Chunnel managed to start at each end and meet in the middle (and we are talking the French and the English here) – *it was amazing.* The Chunnel cost 16 billion to build and it was done in the 1990s using modern technology. Spooners Tunnel was built in 1891 and it was done by two groups – and they met in the middle. Many of the workers were Chinese, Japanese and Italian migrants.

(I imagined the morning briefing: 'Righto chaps. Now you lot, walk 700 big paces, umm, *that* way,' he says, turning slowly about, then thrusting an arm loosely out in one direction. 'You can't understand each other? What's that you say? No, no, I don't speak your language either. But it's okay – we don't need to talk. All you gotta do is put all your gear down there and dig a tunnel back to me'.)

And that's what they did – and they did it with picks and shovels.

I closed my eyes and tried to imagine what it was like to walk in a straight line for 700 metres.

The tunnel was a crucial connection between Nelson and Glenhope for 79 years. The plan was to link Nelson to the West Coast by rail but the connection to the national rail network never happened – it became the 'railway to nowhere'. It was closed in 1955. It was reopened in 2016, after a lot of work, to cyclists and walkers.

At 1.4 kilometres long, it was the longest decommissioned rail tunnel in the Southern Hemisphere. Whatever that meant. *Who came up with these meaningless stats?*

What *was* important, was that I hadn't prepared for this. I'd been a little blasé with regard to lighting on my bicycle. I had a headlamp, somewhere. It was cheap and had fallen apart. I believed it was still onboard, stuffed in one of the panniers. I did have a little torch. In fact, it was so little that it was the same height as Homer – about seven centimetres. It took one AA battery. It was good if it was dark and all you needed it for was to inspect your fingernails.

'How bad can this be?' I wondered.

'Bad,' said Homer.

'No, I mean: "Bad. How *bad* can this be?"', I said. 'It's kind of a rhetorical question. In that, it can't be that bad in bad terms.'

'Whatever,' said Homer. 'But you just used the word bad four times. That sounds pretty bad to me.'

'Mmmnnn,' I considered.

'Can I go leave now?' asked Homer, his voice trembling slightly. 'I don't need to go through this tunnel. I don't do tunnels.'

I went for a distraction: 'Do you know, my good wee mate, that there is a tunnel here in NZ that is named after you? And it's not too far away as the crow flies.'

'Simpson Tunnel,' said Homer and rolled the name around in his mouth to try it for taste. 'I like it,' he declared. 'I know there's a Simpson

Desert in Australia. Simpson was a distinguished name in Ireland. And now a Simpson Tunnel in New Zealand. Ah, whaddaya know. Maybe I do do tunnels. Now where did you say it is?'

I was pleased to see Homer perk up; although there was some name confusion. 'It's not actually called Simpson Tunnel.'

'Oh yeah. Wiseguy eh?' Homer's eyes bulged with agitation. 'Thought you could distract me with some … some distraction. Well it won't work buster.'

'It's called Homer Tunnel, Homer.' I smiled.

Homer squinted suspiciously at me. 'Homer Tunnel, eh. This another one of your cock-and-bull stories?'

'No. No. It's really called Homer Tunnel. But it's over on the way to Milford Sound. It's a monster of a tunnel. Goes right through a mountain.'

'Homer Tunnel you say,' said Homer. 'Well let's go there. Leave this crappy tunnel right here and go through *My* tunnel. Spooner Tunnel *spunnell*. Whoever met a Spooner anyways?'

'Well sure Homey, it could be something we can work on. But right here, right now, Spooner Tunnel is before us and the only way forward.' I didn't want to mention that Spooner Tunnel was actually longer than Homer Tunnel – that pearl of information was also freaking me out a little. Long and dark.

'Mmmn, I'm not sure I should trust you, pal. You haven't been quite up front on this whole trip.' Homer rolled his large eyes downwards. A moment later he rolled them up and gave a loopy grin. 'Look, I may be a bit suspicious … and who could blame me. But this is a great day for me if there truly is a tunnel named in my honour. Who would have thunk? So, I'll cut you some slack on this one but I want to see some good, hard, words on paper evidence – like in a book, telling me about Homer Tunnel – my tunnel. That it's fair dinkum, as an aussie would say. How about that?'

Homer was happy. I was happy; we could move on.

'Look, we will be fine. It's a tunnel. It's got one entrance here, and another opening through there.' I peered deeply into the tunnel. There was no light in the distance. No exit I could see. 'Let's crack on eh mate?'

The tunnel had a curve in it – not a curve to the side but a curve that went slightly up and then down. Its walls were made of tens of thousands of bricks. Amazing workmanship.

There was no way I could ride my bike through it. It was too dark for that. The torch beam was so weak that it couldn't even pool a light in front of me. I found that by shining the light to the side I could use the tunnel wall to navigate. TWDT I named it. Tunnel Wall Directional Technique. If I kept that wall on my right-hand side, then I must be going forward. I had to resist the sensation that made it feel like I was turning a corner; it was nearly overpowering though – the tunnel was taking a sharp turn. But that wasn't possible. Disorientation. Sensibility and using TWDT would get me through. *Use the force, Jedi.*

There's no explaining the dark of a tunnel. It's like being in a cave. It's not a thing, it's a feeling. Like being wrapped in a thick black cloak. Fortunately, I had my torch to keep the cloak at bay.

Halfway through the tunnel, the torch light flickered and went out. The cloak went around me. I was stuck in an inky closet. I was afraid of the dark. Fortunately, this wasn't dark – this was too close for darkness. Darkness needed space. A dark sky is out there, all around you. Tunnel darkness is within you. You are buried alive.

I urgently tapped the torch with my other hand. The light spluttered, then came alive. I knew I only had a moment before it would extinguish again. There was a function on the phone that gave you a light. I scrolled through the phone looking for the app, or whatever the bloody thing was called. Nothing. No symbol that resembled a light. But there would be no panicking in this coffin. I may be buried a hundred metres deep but I wasn't going to panic.

Okay, I was going to panic – but not just yet.

Using the feeble beam, I opened a pannier to search for the broken headlamp. Bananas, socks and other bits fell to the floor of the tunnel.

Wrong pannier. The headlamp was at the bottom of the other pannier. More gear fell to the damp ground.

I put the torch in my mouth, to hold it, and directed the beam onto my shaking hands. I was trying to put the headlamp back together. *Piece of crap, you little piece of crap headlamp.*

It wouldn't work. It was no use. I had no choice but to use the one battery torch and hope it could get the job done. If the worst came to the worst, I could put out my right arm and keeping my hand on the tunnel wall, push on through. Use the wall, with its spider webs, wētāspore and crevices as my sheet of brail – the blind map to lead the blind man forth to everlasting light.

Back near the beginning of the TA, on the ferry from Poutu Point to Helensville, I had escaped the gear nerd and fortuitously ended up on the seat next to Moira. Moira was a bat specialist with DOC. She was a mine of information. I didn't even know NZ had native bats.

Moira schooled me in the ways of bats. Only the short-tailed NZ bat and the vampire bat had adapted to hunting on the ground. They could scuttle along the floor on their wing stumps, scratching their way towards their prey. Or hang motionless on the side of a tunnel wall waiting for the prey to come groping to them.

The exit to the tunnel could finally be seen in the far, *far* distance. A pinprick of light called hope. It grew and grew in size. Light at the end of the tunnel. The little torch did big things that day. It powered itself through Spooners Tunnel.

I found myself gulping for air, like a stranded goldfish, as I exited the tunnel. Someone was lightly sobbing. Was that Homer?

I was in one piece. Homer was in one piece. The bike was in one piece.

The only thing missing was my black peak cap. I kept it strapped to the handlebar bag. It must have come off while I was bumbling about in the dark.

'My hat is missing. We're going to have to go back into the tunnel,' I said.

'No, sweet mother, no!' cried Homer. 'You are insane.'

I smiled coyly. 'Ha, gotcha.' I turned to look back into the deep tunnel. I shuddered. 'Do you seriously think I would go through that again?'

'Your sanity is in question, pal,' said Homer. 'I no longer know what you will do. You've put me in some bad situations on this trip. And there's no escape for me. You've screwed me down. It can't get any worse.'

Little did Homer know.

I began feeling unwell as I rode into Tapawera. My stomach was doing small loops. Perhaps I had over breakfasted. Perhaps I was suffering some post-traumatic stress disorder from Spooners Tunnel. Perhaps I had ingested wētā spore.

The Tapawera café was closed; of course. I should have remembered the theme for this tour: it's either closed or about to close. I bought a large bottle of Primo chocolate milk from the dairy. (Many would consider this to be a make or break move on account of the churning stomach). I wasn't thinking straight. It had been a hell of a morning.

The chocolate milk went down easily enough – but would it stay down? I pedalled steadily up the valley towards Tadmoor. Hops were being grown on both sides of the road. Every field was filled with tall strings of hops vines – acre after acre. I spied some harvesters running down the rows. The hops were trimmed from the wires and fell into long trailers being towed by tractors. Loose cones were sprinkled liberally in the grass on the sides of the road. Houses even had a few vines in the backyard, a bit of home brewing going on. Beer was big business. 350 hectares of hops was grown in NZ in 2013. That was up to 763 in 2019 – and it was growing.

'Did you know, Homer, that Tapawera is the hops capital of NZ?'

'Hops. Mmmmn.' Homer wasn't sure. 'Hops. Is that short for something?'

'No,' I laughed. 'Hops are one of the key ingredients in making beer.'

'Aahhh, beer' sighed Homer. 'Duff. The King of beers.'

'Yes, well, that's debatable,' I replied.

'Oh yeah,' scorned Homer. 'You and your trendy Portland hippy brewsters, with your craft beers (Homer couldn't raise his arms to do the air quotes sign) and micro-breweries. Give me a Duff any day. Mmmn, beer.'

I didn't want a beer. My stomach felt heavy like a stone. I felt like taking a large dump. But where? There were houses regularly along the valley road. There was no bush I could sneak away into. I cycled through a settlement named Kaka – how apt – although that would be spelt Caca. The Kaka Shield was an annual fixture between Tapawera and Richmond, but this was of no concern or help to me.

A young fella on a yellow Suzuki DR650 pulled alongside and loudly enquired if this was the way to the Tadmor Saddle. I confirmed it was. I was pretty sure – but I had never been there himself.

The road turned to gravel and steadily climbed. My stomach turned over. I crested the top at nearly 500 metres and parked the bike. There were fallen pine logs in the bush at the side of the trail. And lots of gorse. I gingerly worked my way through it and found a log suitable to rest my bum against while unburdening. I had an abundance of pine needles to use as toilet paper – just needed to be careful to choose the ones without gorse needles attached.

Nearing Lake Rotoroa, I came across a pop-up café set up in the front yard of a house. An elderly woman was behind the counter. $10 for a cup of Milo and a cheese scone. The price came after the delivery of the goods. The sandflies came after the payment.

'It's going to rain,' commented the woman, smiling as I hopelessly tried to swat the sandflies. 'The sandflies are worst just before it rains.'

The sandflies didn't seem to be bothering her, I noticed. *Probably not sweet enough.*

I sculled the lukewarm drink, pocketed the scone and got out of there before the sandflies finished me. I wasn't in the best of moods. What with tunnel fever, Delhi belly and now a pensioner stealing me blind. She was such a smooth operator and she had my $10 before I knew what had happened – she had probably been stealing the TA'ers blind for years.

Lake Rotoroa was certainly picturesque – and deep – 145 metres to be exact. The sandflies at Lake Rotoroa were described in the guide as 'ferocious'. Stuff that, I thought, I'm out of here. I made for the gravel road leading up to the Braeburn Saddle. A short and nasty climb through brooding beech forest.

Fortunately, the higher elevation meant fewer sandflies. My mood improved by the time I reached the top. It had begun lightly raining – I could manage rain, not sandflies.

It was a fun ride down the 30km to Murchison – the elevation went from 650 metres to 150. The rain was still falling lightly as I made my way to Kiwi Park Motels and Holiday Park. It came highly recommended. However, there were no cabins available – incredible – come on, give me a break.

I ended up in a dumpy motel at the other end of town and I had to cough up $100 for the privilege. Oh, and another $5 for a burst of wifi. (That captive market syndrome again). They had you by the short and curlies – you paid whatever it cost to get inside and away from the sandflies from hell.

The motel had the necessities: hot shower, laundry and kitchen. None of those were in my room, by the way. But I could drag my bike inside, no questions asked, and it was comfortable. It was laundry day; I went back to the office and swiped my ATM card for a bundle of $2 coins. I felt a little wasteful using such a big washing machine for such a small amount of washing – *tant pis,* oh well, I had done two unofficial capitals of NZ that day. Tapawera the hops capital and Murchison the white-water capital. From Murchison, it was a short drive to the many majestic and challenging rivers: the Gowan, Mangles, Matiri, Glenroy,

Matakitaki, Maruia and the renowned Buller. Whitewater nirvana for those into canoeing or kayaking.

Dinner was whatever I could put together from the corner store. By now I was a zen master at mince and rice. Another chance to refine the dish. Spicy Malaysian Curry Big Ben Rice this time.

Murchison to Reefton

72km seal, 50km gravel

It was raining again but only lightly – an English rain, as I mounted up for another day in the saddle. Cattle to round up, steers to brand.

Murchison, huh. What could you say? I laughed: 'There's only two things that come out of Murchison, boy. Steers and Queers. I don't see no horns on you.'

'An Officer and a Gentleman,' said Homer.

'Well, we're not in the middle of nowhere, but we can see it from here.'

'Thelma and Louise,' giggled Homer. 'Good one.'

'You can't handle the truth,' I said. I liked this game.

'A Few Good Men,' said Homer.

The road climbed steadily. It was to be another day of saddle conquering – not the one under my backside however as that pain in the butt was still there – my constant companions still came alive in the afternoons.

'They may take our lives but they'll never take our freedom.'

'Braveheart.'

'Get your stinking paws off me, you damn dirty ape.'

'Planet of the Apes.'

'Ah, you're too good, Homer.'

'Yeah, buddy. That's my world,' said Homer, with a happy sigh. 'Well at least it used to be. Until you dragged me away on this godforsaken trip that we will be lucky to survive.'

Homer reflected: *The Simpsons* had been running since 1989. My lord, he thought. That's more than 30 years. I've raised a family … although, strangely, none of them has grown up – they're not getting any older. Hey, wait a minute – neither am I! Homer needed a beer. Where was the closest Duff brewery? Or a donut. With pink frosting. He was out of his element here but, come to think of it, his 'element' seemed strangely foreign now. Artificial. Was he the same age as DC? Why was he stuck in life? Why was he stuck on these handlebars? Hey pal.'

'Yes, Homer.'

'How old are you?'

'Sixty…ish.'

'How old were you in 1989?'

'Ah, that would be 29.'

'Mmmmn.' Homer paused to think: 'Something's not right.'

'What's the matter?' I asked.

'I don't seem to be getting any older,' quavered Homer. 'Neither is my family. Marge is still the beautiful woman … with the blue poodle on her head. Bart is still 10, Lisa is 8 and Maggie is a baby. She's only one – I think.'

'Yes indeed,' I said. '*The Simpsons* is the longest-running primetime tv series in America.'

'Well, I never,' said Homer.

'It's no wonder you took this sabbatical,' I continued. 'Who wouldn't be burnt out after 32 seasons?'

'C'mon fella,' said Homer, astonished. 'How's that possible? – And what sabbatical?'

'You told me that you had to get out of the U S of A. Coronavirus was out of control. America was a little crazy.'

Homer nodded his head, now recollecting. 'That's right. We had a nut running the place. One day he tried to push the Big Red Button.' Homer shook his head slowly in dismay that someone could be so reckless. 'No, wait a minute. That was me. It was another nut,' yelped Homer. 'We had a nut in the White House. We had a virus running amok. He was trying to build a wall in Mexico. He was blaming everything on China.

His face was getting more and more orange.' Homer hesitated: 'Tell me it's not real.'

'Yes, it's real,' I confirmed. (Now, how could I go about describing this? I had to be delicate.) 'Well, not all of it is real.'

'Okay, which bits?'

'The bit about the nut in The Whitehouse is real – and the nut in the nuclear plant.' I took it carefully. 'The bit about you not aging is also real. You are the same age as when you started in *The Simpsons* in 1989.' I tried to steer the conversation. *You are a plastic doll – you're a goddam cartoon.* No, I couldn't scream those. 'Umm, you're very lucky.'

'Lucky, schmucky,' said Homer.

'All that you know, is at the end.'

'The Silver Surfer,' said Homer.

'Come on, Homey,' I soothed. 'We've had a couple of moments, true. But nothing bad will happen to you. I will look after you.'

The gravel was wet and heavy. I had to go down a gear to keep moving. A hard slog – the gravel was syrupy and clung to the sides of the tyres. A steady headwind had also sprung up. All in all, it was turning into a slugfest. I hunkered down and dug in. I was strong. 'Go ahead, make my day.'

'Dirty Harry,' said Homer.

I noted the uncommon number of bridges I was crossing. Ah, *The Bridges of Madison County* was a film about grand covered bridges in that county. A National Geographic photographer was documenting them. The real story was about the temptation between the photographer, the handsome Robert, and Francesca, a woman living a dull life on a local farm. I smiled, remembering. Mostly remembering how the music built and built to a crescendo – much like the affair.

The perilous affair burnt rapidly. They couldn't continue and the parting was wretched. The separation tore hearts both on screen and off. I had felt destitute for days.

'The human heart has a way of making itself large again even after it's been broken into a million pieces.'

'Bridges of Madison County,' replied Homer. 'And why are you sobbing?'

'What? – Not,' I said, clumsily wiping a tear. 'I swallowed a moth. I'm a little chokey; that's all.'

The Maruia Saddle was 580 metres high. I did it fine but it was hard going on that wet gravel. This was one of the days when you just needed to do the business. Stopping for a break wasn't pleasant either. Bumble bees would instantly descend. Where did they come from? What do they want? I couldn't work it out. I'd never been bombarded by bumble bees before – it wasn't friendly. They could probably give a warm furry feeling – with a sting in the tail. It was 50km of wet gravel before I again hit the seal.

Springs Junction had a café that was open. It was more like a roadside diner. More like what I've been after the whole trip, I reckoned, as I wearily leant the bike against a table outside.

The young Indian fella behind the counter proudly said they were open until 7pm, seven days a week.

'Now that's what I'm talking about,' I said, joyfully.

'Napoleon Dynamite,' said the young Indian.

'Could be,' I said. 'A large omelette and a vanilla milkshake, please.'

'No problem,' said the young man.

'And I will follow that milkshake with another milkshake.'

'So that will be two milkshakes.'

'Yes. But not at the same time,' I said carefully, wanting to get this right. 'One vanilla milkshake, followed sometime later by another vanilla milkshake.'

I was knackered. The gravel had taken it out of me. I had hit a bit of a wall. I took a seat at the table. The America's Cup regatta was on the telly in the corner. Pictures being beamed in from Auckland harbour – I felt a million miles away.

The omelette wasn't really an omelette: it was more like a pancake. The cook didn't really have the omelette thing down, with the folding over and all. But to me it was a magnificent culinary masterpiece. Three eggs and large. The protein boost of eggs and milk went straight to the muscles and I was charged. Ready to take on the mean 250-metre climb to the Rahu Saddle.

This part of NZ was dominated by saddles. How bizarre, how bizarre.

'OMC,' said Homer.

I pulled strongly all the way to the top; God bless protein. The TA Official Guide described the downhill from the Rahu saddle, as one that just kept giving. And it did. What a ride down into Reefton. It had been a big day but satisfying to knock the bugger off.

I had digs at a former flatmate's place. She had a sense of humour that was very west coast. I found the head of a Merino ram in the bed.

The Godfather.

Reefton

Day off

My former flatmate, Helen, looked after me well – aside from putting the ram's head in my bed. She fed and watered me and recharged my batteries. My knee enjoyed the day off – the rest of the body was remarkably pain free. I had done a few stretches early on in the tour but that practice had fallen by the wayside.

Reefton was probably the only town on the west coast that had done well during Covid-19. It had experienced a steady flow of NZ tourists.

Reefton was the first town in the Southern Hemisphere to get electricity. And, just quietly, it needs it, I thought. The place attracted dark clouds like a dentist attracted teeth. The forbidding hills gave it a funereal air. Its main street fought valiantly against the atmosphere. Brightly painted shopfront facades were a grand idea. They uplifted spirits and combined with some quirky names to give the town a real character. The Reefton Coffin Co and the Quaint and the Curious, just a couple. Down the side streets were The School of Mines, Oddfellows Hall and the Reefton Masonic Hall.

Reefton was a thriving gold mining town in the late 19th century. It had done well to adapt.

Helen's sister, Margaret, gave me a send-off with a lamb dinner that evening. (That was lamb spelt with an L. Not an R). I did the carving of the meat – I went against the grain – my way of life.

Reefton to Ikamatua

8km seal, 15km gravel, 33km rough track

I reluctantly dragged myself out of the big, warm bed. I went through the centuries-old male ritual of scratching, rubbing, stretching and groaning. I plucked the guide off the bedside table: The Big River Track. TA Official Guide: This 5 to 7-hour stage is challenging. If it's been raining, check at the I-Site to see if it's still passable. If not, then bypass along Highway 7.

It had rained a couple of days earlier, but the track was passable for all entrants in this year's TA. Some days were going to be wetter than others but this track was always wet. It ran up a river and through swamp and rainforest; water was its blood.

I suspected the majority of TA'ers this year would bypass Big River on account of its reputation. Not because it was too wet. I was a belligerent fool much of the time but I was also an adventurer. Had been my whole life. I liked to put myself in places where adventures could occur – you couldn't organise an adventure. An adventure was a spontaneous happening. But you could put yourself in a position, with enough time, for an adventure to be likely.

I hadn't planned on an adventure involving a large dog who obviously wanted to tear me apart. Getting out of small towns in NZ could often involve running a gauntlet of a town's mutts. Usually, they were just yappy little hounds. The Reefton dog on duty early that morning was a brindle Mastiff crossed with something nasty. It stormed along the front of a house yard as I rode by. Fortunately, it was behind a fence.

I was counting on it being confined to that property because if this huge brute got loose it could do some damage. I didn't think I could outrun it – wrong bike setup for sprinting.

The dog bounded straight through to the neighbour's property.

I felt a sense of precognition – an extrasensory perception – What would HST say in this moment?: 'Fear is a healthy instinct, not a sign of weakness.' Or: 'Pray to God, but row away from the rocks.'

'Geez, Wayne', I prayed. There was no fence between the neighbours. The monster dog was still restrained behind the roadside fence though. I tried to power up on the bike. The dog sailed across onto the next neighbour's property. It looked even angrier now, if that was possible. I was able to get a good long look at it as we were now spending time together. It had bloodshot eyes and drool was spraying from its great slavering jaws.

A fence on the corner pulled it up short, fortunately for me, and I was able to perform a wobbly escape down the road.

I've been mentally preparing myself for Big River, not to be torn apart by a lion, I breathed. That was my reservoir of adrenalin run dry for the day.

The challenge began only one kilometre from Reefton. Gravel and a climb up the aptly named Devil's Creek Valley. At 10km the track went to 4WD.

There were two signs at this point. The newer sign said:

WARNING (in large red letters)
This road is not maintained past this point
and is not suitable for any vehicles.
Any persons proceeding do so at their OWN risk.

The sign had been peppered with gunshot and I couldn't tell if the sign said person or persons as it looked like a shotgun had been used on that sentence.

There was another, older, sign.

It said: Road Closed. Use at own risk.

The signs were in bad shape, but you got the message. Not for Sunday walkers.

It was 25km to the Big River Hut. It was also a 550-metre climb. I toiled away in bottom gear up the track, which had deep ruts and loose rock. This was the toughest climbing I had done on the tour. The Maungatapu was steeper but Big River was gnarlier. It was only just rideable for me and required short, grunty spurts of energy to get over obstacles. I did walk in a couple of places.

The constant hum of wasps accompanied me. But zero bird noise. Curious.

It took me four hours to do the 25km to the hut. There were three river crossings just before the hut. You could bypass them by taking a cycle track along the river bank. To hell with that, I thought. I've come this far. I'm having a go. I made only one of them without touching down.

Thus, I arrived at Big River Hut with wet feet but a full heart. That was fun. Big River was originally a gold mining town. There was little evidence left behind.

The hut was set on a glorious abutment overlooking the river. It appeared to be a newish hut and was in great shape, spic and span. There was a modern long drop, well vented. The hut had running water. It had three rooms, it catered for a lot of people. I had it all to myself.

I took my shoes and socks off and laid them outside to dry. Fat chance. The sun was out but it was a lukewarm orb. I put a brew on and dug out the sandwich I had bought that morning in Reefton – and a large slice of chocolate cake. Food and drink tasted so much better when you were pushing the body.

The visitor's book made for interesting reading. Luigi had been through the day before. He looked to have hooked up with another wingman. Well, wingwoman – he had gone the batgirl route.

Good boy. Luigi had taken the hard option of doing Big River rather than bypassing on the road – 'chicken run' – as it was called. Luigi had taken on all three of the hard options on the TA. Proper. Luigi had tested his mettle and found that he was made of the right stuff. He had true grit.

There were other names in the book that I recognised. Those that I'd been cycling with on the first few days in Northland. Some of them were now nearly a week ahead of me. Still, I had taken four rest days from the tour – and yes, I was slow.

The Waiuta Track Boardwalk was a grand feat of trail building. It ran for some distance from below Big River Hut and led to the Waiuta-Big River Track. The term track could be used loosely as initially it followed a stream bed. No chance of me riding this section. It was a lot of pushing and lifting to get my bike up the rock ledges and over the fallen branches. Would be fun on an unladen, full suspension mountain bike. Better still, my e-bike.

The bush was sopping wet; I suspected this was typical. I leant against a bank and found my sleeve instantly sodden.

The track was wet and muddy. I suspected – no, I knew – it could get worse. There hadn't been a lot of rain the past few days. If it bucketed down it could become unpassable: the streams could become raging torrents and quickly. The TA was fortunate this year to have the Big River track available.

The track was slippery and off camber in parts. There were huge drops on the left-hand side. I didn't want to look too closely but a couple of times I took a quick peek to see what was over there. Nothing, really, but air. There were beech trees valiantly clinging to the slopes. I hoped I could grab one of those if I found myself falling. Better to beware. This was definitely the most technically challenging day of the TA.

The trail ducked into gulches and then climbed steeply out. It required a heads-up approach and forward planning. All necessary skills when dirt biking or mountain biking. Decisions had to be made quickly.

I had done a couple of dirt bike courses with NZ Enduro legend, Chris Birch.

Birchy told us to identify the danger, then look up to where the good stuff was on the track. Where you could find traction. Then head for that. The bike would take care of the dangerous bit. Acknowledge it, then ignore it.

I was also acutely aware that I was alone. If I got into trouble here it could go west in a hurry. Or was that east? Homer was going to be of little use. My tracker device did have an emergency function. Apparently, you could push the button on the left and it would signal you were in trouble – or was that the one on the right? The buttons were so worn that I couldn't make out what their function was. Besides, the tracker had proved less than reliable to this point. I doubted it was capable of bringing in a chopper full of paramedics to save the day.

I elected to walk a few particularly perilous looking corners. There was still plenty of excitement to be had on the trail without upping the risk. Tree roots forked off at crazy angles. Combining the wet roots with an off-camber track made for some hectic action. I found myself sliding in full speedway mode a couple of times. Mercifully I slid into a bank each time.

It did eventually turn to custard. I got into a slide into a tight corner. I tried desperately to unclip my foot from the pedal but the shoe cleat was so damaged from walking that it refused to let go.

The back wheel slid off the edge of the track and I found myself falling backwards. *Oh Lordy Lordy*. I prayed it was a short drop, not a precipice.

I had been in this situation before. On the Old Ghost Rd. I had been clipped in then. I had no luggage on the bike on that trip but had been wearing a heavyish backpack. I had made a small mistake on a rocky ledge and bounced backwards. The weight of the pack, and not being able to unclip in time, had found me falling backwards over a drop. That had been a decent one. It had resulted in cuts and bruises and a broken wrist.

Funny, the thoughts you could have while falling. Like crashing in a car, or on a motorbike – I had done plenty of those. I marvelled at the way time appeared to stand still. You could think about all sorts of things; it was quite pleasant. You were sort of floating in an embryonic fluid. Then, 'whammo': things suddenly got real. I may have been an 'expert faller' but it didn't get easier. In fact, as I got older the falls seemed more significant. They were still just as surprising and bone jarring as when I was younger. When I was young I used to spring to my feet as soon as I stopped sliding or tumbling, then run back and check to see if the bike was okay. Nowadays I lay for a while. Worked my fingers a bit – moved the arms. Then quietly waggled the legs. If all of those parts were co-operating, I would gradually roll over and pull myself onto all fours. I knew the way up from there.

If one could just capture that mid-crash sensation – the freefall – put that in a bottle: ha, that was just around the corner with the advent of the virtual reality world. My avatar would be riding this one out and I would be tucked up on the La-Z-Boy, VR headset on, stuffing my face full of chips and dip and dribbling with glee at the tragedy unfolding. I was having all of these pleasant thoughts as I fell and wondered just how bad this was going to be.

I fell backwards a couple of metres into an assemblage of rotten punga and soft ferns. I lay there for a moment to see if any pain registered. Nope. I could waggle my fingers and toes. *I may have gotten away with this one.*

The bike was lying upside down on top of me. I was still cleated in. *Great work, cleats.*

It took some manoeuvring to get out from under the bike. Then to drag it back up onto the track. I had no injuries; not a scratch. The bike appeared undamaged. The Aero carrier needed pulling around to straighten the panniers, but it was fine. The panniers had even stayed securely onboard. Now, *that* was a test of equipment. No lab testing – this was the real deal.

I had dodged a bullet – fortune smiled on the brave. I mounted up and prepared to venture forth. It was then that I looked down and noticed Homer. Homer's left arm was in two pieces. The lower part of his arm was hanging by a thread.

'Ummm,' I ventured. 'Does that hurt?'

'Does what hurt?' replied Homer. 'Yes, the fact that you tried to *kill* me, hurts.'

'Sorry about that,' I apologised. 'Bit of an error.' I peered closely at Homer. Homer's expression hadn't changed. It still looked bewildered and his eyes were bugging off into the distance. His normal demeanour – his look.

'You have no pain anywhere?' I enquired.

'Nope, all good, pal. But don't pull that stunt again.'

'Umm, your arm seems to be in two pieces,' I said, casually; trying to sound non-alarmist.

There was a moment of quiet.

'Dulp'. Then reality set in. 'Oh my god! What have you done to me?' screamed Homer. 'You've mutilated me. Help, help!'

'I'm not sure it's that bad,' I said, calmly.

'My arm has fallen off, you idiot – how much worse could it be!'

'Let me see what I can find to fix this,' I said, scrounging in the left pannier to find the tool bag.

'Should I pray?' said Homer, in a frail voice. 'Am I going. I'm going. I'm going. I can feel it, I'm slipping away. Hey! Why is there no blood?'

I found a small roll of duct tape. Here was another delicate Homer question to be circumnavigated: 'It's the altitude, Homer, the blood congeals immediately.'

I fashioned a silver sling. 'There, you look like a proper adventurer now,' I said, satisfied with my medical skills.

'Adventurer schmenturer,' replied Homer. 'Easy for you to say. If you're such an adventurer, why aren't you wearing a sling?'

'Good point, Homey. But one of us has to ride the bike.'

'Cut the Homey. I obviously took the impact. Saved us. Kept your sorry arse alive, pal. You can thank me later.'

'Thanks Homer.'

'Don't mention it. Now let's get the hell out of these woods.'

Ikamatua was like an oasis after the hectic day in Big River. I went straight to the Ikamatua Hotel – it had camping and cabins. I so wanted a cabin. A cabin was available, hallelujah. And it only cost $30 – what a place. I left my muddied bike outside the cabin and went next door to the Ikamatua Store. The girl behind the counter took one look at me and laughed.

'You've just come off Big River,' she shouted.

'Yes, how can you tell?'

'Look at the state of you,' she bellowed. 'They either come in here muddied or bloodied.'

'I did try for a bit of both,' I admitted. 'I got a bit lucky today.'

'Okay, tell me,' she smiled, and leaned forward. 'You hated it. You're never going to do it again.'

'No, I loved it,' I said. 'It was definitely tricky but it was very cool.'

She laughed again, loudly. 'I reckon only about 20 percent of the TA riders like Big River. The rest hate it and will never do it again.'

'Yeah, well I'm not sure how many actually attempt it,' I agreed. 'I reckon they should all have a go. It's part of the TA. Even if you end up walking it all. So what? At least you did it.'

There were a few others in the store but no one seemed interested in our conversation, or the fact that the young woman was bellowing at me. She must be hard of hearing, I thought.

I went to the shelves to find some chips to celebrate my survival. I noted the array of magazines on the shelf. There weren't many but there was a common theme: *NZ Hunter*, *Hunting New Zealand*, *Rod and Rifle*, *NZ Hunting* and *Wildlife*.

A shopper went to the counter and shouted something at the young lady. She shouted back. They shouted amiably to one another about the weather, the day and whatever else they could think of, that would be worth shouting about.

Peculiar, I thought, as I purchased some chips and, of course, a milkshake.

Outside the store, there were a couple of trucks pulled up. The drivers, a man and a woman, were shouting at each other about the day's driving – they were only a metre apart.

Must be a lot of noise, here on the west coast, I considered, as I trudged back to my cabin. People were deaf from it. Perhaps, all the banging of pickaxes and coal box carts in the mines. The detonating of hillsides. The gunfire.

I sat on the chair outside my cabin. I munched my way happily through the chips and slurped merrily on the milkshake. My bike stood muddy and unbowed by the wall. *What a day.* I finished the chips, popped the bag with gusto and headed for the pub.

The publican was a busy man. He not only tended to those sitting around the bar, he had to run the campground as well. He wasn't flustered though. He appeared to have just the one speed – medium, you could call it. He too, had a particularly loud way of talking. He shouted to all and sundry around the bar. They shouted back. It was a grand time.

He had a beard, probably requisite for a publican on the coast. He gave me some coins for the laundry. For free. He also showed me where a hose and brush were to wash my bike. And where the well-stocked kitchen was. Cooking gear, crockery and a bewildering array of cutlery; incredible. He shouted at me to just help myself to whatever I needed, and if I needed anything, to just give him a shout.

I thought I might just park up there – for the rest of my life. $30 for a cabin. It was small. It had only a single bed. But it was spotless and nicely painted. It even had a bible in the side table. A free laundry. A kitchen. A store next door that sold milkshakes. People were so nice.

$30 for the night. I would have stayed there for the rest of his life, but I didn't think I could stand all the shouting, even if they did mean well.

The two young women, doing the South Island portion of the TA, rolled into the Ikamatua Hotel back yard. They had bypassed the Big River section. They set up their tents in the large grassed area. I noticed, with curiosity, that they set up their tents a considerable distance from each other. Not a good sign. Only a few days into the trip and they weren't playing friends anymore.

One of them informed me that they'd bought their tents specifically for the TA and they were determined to use them as much as possible. I said there were cabins available and they were great, and cheap. She said that her friend was a snorer and she couldn't share a cabin with her – and that was why they set their tents some distance apart.

I cleaned Big River off my bike and did my ablutions. I changed into my spare shorts, put on my spare shirt and put all my dirty gear into the washing machine. Then it was time to eat – in a pub. Pub food. Meat and three veg. Proper.

I considered the laminated menu. There was fish and chips – cod – they were on the West Coast. Bangers and mash. Tripe. I gave a small shudder. My mother used to cook tripe – and brains, sweetbreads – all those things they cooked in those days when you didn't have much money. The last time I had tripe was when I visited my dad in the retirement home. I had tried to pretend it was calamari.

'I will have the lamb shanks,' I said, to the publican, who was also the waiter. But not the cook.

'Good choice, if I don't say so,' shouted the publican. 'Will that be one or two lamb shanks?'

'Two thanks,' I replied, feeling so good. What a day this had turned into. I could be upside down at the bottom of a gully. But no, I was in the Ikamatua Hotel being offered lamb shanks.

'Okay, that will be three lamb shanks,' said the publican, loudly.

'No, just the two,' I corrected.

'Well two is really three,' smiled the publican.

'Oh, is it?' I said, with some confusion.

'Yes, you see they're small ones.' The publican beamed at me as if he'd just told me that pigs could fly. 'So, if you order two, you get three.'

'Ah, I see,' I said. And I did. 'Righto, make it three.'

'Good. That will be two then,' shouted the publican, and marched away happy.

The lamb shanks duly arrived and there were two.

Ikamatua to Kumara

56km seal, 28km cycle trail

Ikamatua was a tough place to leave. It had all the amenities to make a man happy. I had noticed wood chips spread liberally about the back yard of the pub. They were from the previous weekend's wood chopping event. The whiff of two-stroke gas. Stihl, Husqvarna, McCulloch chainsaws wailing into the wind. This was real man's country.

I got away early, before the shouting began. It was setting up to be a nice day. The sun was on my back as I pedalled away.

There were two roads that followed the Grey River down to Greymouth. I chose the one on the north side – the road less travelled. The south side was Highway 7 and it was busy, with plenty of trucks working it. I could have detoured up a road to visit Blackball and the infamous, Formerly the Blackball Hilton – a historic hotel built in the early 1900's. In the 1990's it was renamed the Blackball Hilton. This caused repercussions with a certain hotel chain overseas. Hence, the Formerly being stuck in there.

I bypassed it and carried straight on to Greymouth. I ran the gauntlet of Highway 6 for the last few k's into Greymouth. No shoulder and trucks – yuck.

'Hey, Homer, how's the arm?' I enquired, as I rode into town.

'Mmmn, warm. It's so cosy in its little silver blanky,' said Homer. 'I could almost think it's not broken. But it is!' He paused a moment: 'Strangely, I feel no pain.'

No shit, Sherlock. 'Homer, do you know I raced here, in this town? I reckon Greymouth might be the coolest street race in NZ now, with the demise of Paeroa.'

'No, I don't. I don't know a thing about you – aside from the fact that you abducted me – like those aliens did. Then you played mind games with me and took me to dark places, like …, like …'

'Like nightime, Homer.'

'Yes, exactly like nightime. You went inside my head and took my brain,' bawled Homer. 'Now I have no memory. How did I get here?'

'Don't you remember when we met?' I prompted. 'In the Bin Inn, Whangārei.'

'I think so,' replied Homer, dreamily. 'The place with all the candy floss, Milk Duds, Jolly Ranchers – and socks.'

'No,' I said. 'I'm not sure where that was. I found you on a shelf in Bin Inn. You were between the Lentils and the Alfalfa.'

'Aagh, Alfa!' screeched Homer. 'I would never… I only drive American. Why you little …'

'Anyways,' I interrupted. 'I dusted you off, and put you in with my quinoa and polenta.'

Homer puzzled, 'Do I even know those women?'

'Ha,' I laughed. 'I was trying some alternative foods, shall we say.' I nodded. 'But, it's alright. I'm back on course now.'

I had raced the Greymouth Motorcycle Street Race just the once, a few years before. It was a quick track, I recalled – through the main streets of the town. I was curious to compare how the streets looked when prepared for racing as opposed to being readied for a normal shopping day. No deer fencing on the edge of the footpath this day – or hay bales on the corners and strapped to lampposts. It wasn't often you could say you raced your bike past a police station – legally.

The police station was on Guinness St. Guinness St connected with Tainui St which was home to Revingtons Hotel. It was here that a woman had a Saturday night on the town, arriving by horse. Her teetering outside Revingtons attracted attention from the patrons. She took this as a cue to offer rides around the town's centre. The police took this as a cue to investigate the equine activity. She was warned to go home. However, she refused, claiming there were no laws preventing people riding horses in the West Coast township and she was going to continue with the fun.

'She was a little intoxicated but she was in control,' said one patron. 'She was leading the horse, just walking on the footpath – and had a high-vis jacket on. The young ones were enjoying it. People thought it was cool.'

The police did not think it was 'cool'. Officers pulled her from the saddle to arrest her for being drunk and disorderly on a horse.

'She tried to bring the horse into the hotel's reception to avoid them,' said another onlooker. 'It was possible the woman tried to get the horse to kick the police and run them down.'

She was let off with a warning and given her horse back.

I chose the café I had used in previous visits – The Bonzai Café. I preferred to call it the Banzai Café. More in keeping with racing. I leant my bike against the back of a wrought iron seat on the footpath. It was outside the café – I could keep half an eye on it. The Bonzai served a good milkshake. An omelette followed and a huge cheese scone for later.

It was good to be back by the sea. It was a vigorous West Coast swell; filled with contagious energy.

'So, let me get this straight,' said Homer, as I readied the bike. 'You found me in a store.'

'Yep, I took you home and a week later we started the Tour Aotearoa. And here we are now – the time of our lives.'

'Okay, I'm willing to forget the kidnapping – for the moment,' said Homer, reasonably. 'But why are you on this trip? What's in it for you?'

'Ah …'

'Midlife crisis, eh, Pal.' Homer hesitated for a minute. Then his brow furrowed – or it would have, if it weren't made of yellow plastic. He blurted, 'I may never have one of those – I may never get old enough.'

I didn't know how to comfort Homer, so I stuck to my own story. 'Not really a crisis,' I said. 'My life has been a series of happy mini-crises. I like to call them adventures. My children have left home … I'm hoping they don't grow up – at least, don't settle down. That's a state of mind, in my books. I'm looking for things I can do that push me a bit. I've discovered that I have some masochistic attraction to things that make me uncomfortable.'

'Oh. So you're like some crazy daredevil,' said Homer. 'Like that dude, what's his name – Bear Grylls.'

'Ha, no. Not at all. I'm no daredevil.' I mused: 'I just like it when it gets a bit gnarly – difficult. Must be the Scottish genes. More likely, the Irish genes,' I joked. 'I actually don't really plan my life. If something seems like a good idea, I do it. Even if it's a good idea I've only had three minutes ago and will take three years to complete. Away I go.'

'And here we are,' agreed Homer.

'Yep, here we are. This was one of those "good ideas",' I confirmed. 'A mate, Taito, is on this very TA. He's probably a week ahead. He told me he was doing it – so I signed up. That's all.'

'Oh, Mr Airhead. Duncan the Dummy. So if your mate said jump off the bridge you would do it?'

'No. Well, perhaps.'

I pedalled up onto the Greymouth stop bank beside the river mouth. This was the beginning of the West Coast Wilderness Trail. No more having to deal with Kiwi drivers for a couple of days. *Yeah baby.*

The trail was very easy cycling. It was a very cruisy day. I probably should have pushed a little harder, gone a little further, but I couldn't find a reason to. I had long ago lost that racy feeling I had felt at the beginning of the TA.

My trip then, had been a two-dimensional journey. I had found the third dimension on the road to Damascus – that would be the road from Martinborough.

The trail turned inland at Kumara Junction and I found myself in Kumara, a quirky village with only a few hundred residents. In 1876 gold was discovered nearby and Kumara took off. It was also the home of Richard Seddon who became Prime Minister in 1893. The Coast to Coast endurance race began each year from Kumara Beach. There was no giant kumara in Kumara.

I rolled into the Greenstone Retreat. There was no one about – a note on the door of the villa said to help yourself and the boss would be back later. Nice.

The retreat had a hippy feeling to it. Handcrafted doors and fittings carved from native woods. Hanging crystals and leadlight windows. Soothing music and incensed aromas infused the retreat.

I wouldn't have been surprised to find Jimi Hendrix playing in the back yard and muslin dressed hippies dancing in the rain; it had that kind of vibe.

Well, I would have been a little surprised – and it wasn't raining.

The boss arrived a little later and gave me a run down on the place and how it worked. There were no rooms available but there was a bunkroom with no one booked into it. I could take a bunk. The price was right, but, what if a snorer arrived and took the bunk opposite? That incessant sawing melody of the terminal snorer that could tear into your very soul and destroy your world. I would have no choice but to stuff a pillow over their face until the snoring ceased. I chose instead to set up my tent in a far corner of the property.

A bearded, long haired, earnest looking young man arrived. He was barefoot and going for hippy sheik with his look – a white Jesus. I had met plenty of his sort when I lived in Vermont, USA. The more 'hippy' they appeared, the more likely they were to be on a trust fund from Daddy's New York bank account. The dude went straight for a herbal tea.

'Gidday, mate,' I said.

'Hello,' said the fake hippy, looking all about but not at me.

A stunning conversation could have been about to break out: not. However, we were interrupted by the arrival of the two young South

Island TA cyclists that I had kept bumping into since the ferry crossing of the Cook Strait.

'Are you stalking me?' I asked them.

'No,' they replied emphatically, in unison.

Ha, irony wasted on the youth.

The fake hippy navigated away from me and towards the young women. They caught his current and drifted towards him. *He's probably named Eddie*. I watched with dull amusement as the attraction ritual began. So predictable.

I switched my attention to the amenities which were nice and everything was there that could make your stay comfortable. There was even massage offered. I decided to try to shift modes – to go in search of my cool daddy inner zen. I booked a massage.

The massage room had crystals, incense burning and meditative music piping through. *What else would you expect?* The massage therapist said she had just returned from collecting greenstone in a river nearby.

Oh well. I might not have much in common with this crowd but they are nice enough. If she could just work some relief into my legs, it would be a beautiful thing.

The massage therapist said she had treated many TA riders in the past week. She also said that she was no good at riding a bicycle. But she did like to ride motorbikes.

What?

She liked nothing better than to roost up a fine stretch of gravel track. The massage room soon became a hot bed of discussion on the merits of two-stroke versus four-stroke. The best trails thereabouts and what tyres to use in the mud. She did get a bit excited a couple of times and gripped my calf like it was a rubber throttle. I gave a little squeal – which she took as encouragement.

The Theatre Royal Café and Restaurant, in the main street of Kumara, was a hint posh for me. I hardly had clothes for fine dining.

Prospectors Fish and Chips was more the go. It was set up in a bright orange caravan at the far end of the village. A funky little set up offering fresh local food and an interesting menu. I rung my order through from the Greenstone Retreat. I opted for the goat burger but no, it was no longer on the menu. A beef burger and kumara fries instead.

I cycled to the takeaway caravan. The paddock beside the caravan had several goats grazing in it; still alive. *Ha*

I took my meal back to the retreat. The young women were by now totally enraptured in the false hippy's groove and were well locked into his current. They didn't even acknowledge my presence on the next table – despite my being a fellow TA'er. *Reality check, old timer.*

Kumara to Ross

24km seal, 17km gravel, 64km cycle trail

Was the mattress getting narrower or was it my imagination? I enjoyed tenting but my high-tech mattress wasn't cutting the mustard. I had lost a few kilos in weight so I certainly wasn't getting bigger. I couldn't roll over without falling off the bloody thing. Night was a time for sleeping, not concentrating on maintaining a position on the beam – it wasn't yoga. The mattress took 20 puffs to fill. I did it in two sets of 10 to save myself from passing out. It was comfortable enough; just. It just wasn't wide enough. An elite athletic bike packer probably had some hover-rotate move to turn over on the mattress without tipping off. I more resembled a sea lion recently beached. A rollover for me was a laden whole body commitment, not some whimsical gesticulation.

I also wished for a proper pillow. I was using a bag liner stuffed with clothes as a pillow. Perhaps I was getting soft.

Then there were the roosters. One started up at 3am. Another started shortly after, in competition. The first one was hitting the perfect, 'Cockadoodle doodle.' The second was in such a hurry to catch up it was slurring its doodle. More a, 'Cockadurdle durdle'. *Who in their right mind keeps roosters?*

The Wilderness Trail was in great shape. A lot of money was spent in maintaining it. It was one of the most popular trails on the NZ cycle trails network. It was up there with the Otago Rail Trail. I chatted briefly with three women who were doing it on e-bikes. Their husbands were setting up camp at Hans Bay, on the shores of Lake Kaniere. They had those boys well trained.

The Kapitea Reservoir, with its mountain backdrop, was stunning. Blackened tree stumps poked from the water. A shag perched on a tall trunk. The lake was known locally as Dillmans Dam. It was man-made and covered two-and-a-half kilometres in area. It was part of the Duffers/Dillman/Kumara Hydroelectric Power Scheme that powered the West Coast. The scheme first generated power in 1928.

An intake in the Kawhaka Creek diverted up to 12 cumecs (cubic metres per second) into the Kawhaka Race for use by the Duffers Power Station. Water discharged into Loopline Lake – sometimes called Kumara Reservoir – and in turn, into Kapitea Lake. An intake on the short dam of this lake fed up to 10 cumecs through the Dillmans Power House into a 1.8-kilometre canal, then through the Kumara Power House, before liberating it to the Taramakau River.

The water was then funnelled onto a paddle wheel powered by two local beavers – who only worked for carrots – and it spilled alarmingly into a pond where it was aerated by the flapping wings of 1000 pink flamingos. *Just kidding.*

There were water races and outlets at nearly every turn. The water appeared to me to be flowing uphill when I was riding down and, conversely, to be flowing downhill when I was pedalling up. I was enchanted – and a little bamboozled. It was time to push on, and quickly; my pride wouldn't let me be overtaken by some 'café cruisers' – even if they were on e-bikes.

The bush grew close beside the track – ancient Podocarp forest pressed in until I reached an opening and a sprawling suspension bridge.

Cowboy Paradise was nearby. The mock 'Wild West Town' had become a feature of the Wilderness Trail – for better or for worse. It was run by a chap who had become a dubious star of Facebook. There were probably more descriptions of him to be found than Wyatt Earp. He was an acquired taste and it usually depended on which day you came across him, or even, which hour.

The place was staffed by young attractive women from foreign countries. Usually woofers although, with Covid about, a ready supply of woofers probably wasn't available. The staff were regularly turned over due to factors beyond my knowledge. I suspected that a young lady in paradise would have to keep one eye over her shoulder and getting out of Dodge could become urgent at some point.

The TA guide noted that Cowboy Paradise had accommodation and food, (including the world's most expensive frozen pies). The young foreigners this day offered me a toasted sandwich and a cup of tea for a king's ransom. That captive market syndrome again. And cash only.

I remembered the place as being a bit of a shithole last time I'd visited. Crap lying about – unfinished projects. Piles of timber – abandoned machinery. It appeared to have gone even further backwards.

It did have saloon swinging doors. A feeble nod to the wild west. Apart from that, it probably should be renamed Cowboy Shithole, I reckoned, as I rode away. What was The Eagles line?: 'Call someplace paradise, kiss it goodbye.'

It was a really fantastic zig-zag ride from Cowboy Paradise. Weka were about and one was so friendly it investigated my bike in close detail when I stopped at a gate. It was downhill and stellar riding beside the Lake Kaniere Water Race.

The trail then ducked into native bush – you could take the sealed road running parallel to the track if you were in a hurry. There was a stop bank trail beside the Hokitika River and this led to Hokitika township.

Hokitika was the centre of the West Coast gold rush in the 1800s. Historic buildings abounded. However, I wasn't sticking around, I was crunching kilometres.

My bike, the Giant XTC 29er, was still going strong. I was surprised at how well it was going with little maintenance – *okay, no maintenance*. My brother-in-law, Murray, was a bike guru and he was even more surprised than me. We had a phone conversation, back when I was in Ikamatua, basically about the Big River track.

'When did you get the hub on that Giant replaced?' asked Murray.
'Not,' I replied.
'What do you mean, "not"?', said Murray.
'Not.'
'You're a not.'
'No, you're a not.'
'You're a not.'
'No, you're a not.'
'Not.'
'Not.'
'Well I'm glad we got that sorted,' said Murray.
'Me too,' I chuckled.
'The Shimano hubs on those bikes are notorious for blowing up,' said Murray. 'I can't believe it's gone that far.'
'Well …,' I considered. 'I'm glad you told me that *after* Big River. Fortunately, I've only got a couple more hills before Bluff. She'll be right.'
'Not.'

I put a little lube on the chain each morning. That was it. I was careful when changing down gears and made sure to ease up the pedal stroke – take the weight off the gear train. The bike had taken a bit of a pounding down some of the slopes, but nothing like a normal downhill on a fully suspended mountain bike without luggage. I had broken one spoke on the rear – to save it flopping about I had it cable tied to its neighbour.

The bike had little use before I bought it. The previous owner had bought it new; it would have been an expensive bike then – purchased with great unfulfilled intention. I considered the bike to be in better shape than I was.

The trail from Hokitika to Ross rivalled the Hauraki Rail Trail in its rating on the boredom scale. It was still part of the Wilderness Trail and it was formerly a rail trail. Dead straight, flat and monotonous – innate fundamentals for a decent railway line. Ideal podcast country. I met only one other cyclist on it – a man who was going in the same direction – quicker obviously as he caught me. The man was also wearing ear buds and listening to a podcast. We shouted at each other for a few minutes about our respective journeys. The man commuted each day on this mindless stretch to get to work. He lived in Ross. He had done the TA a couple of years before; he loved to cycle. We should have removed our ear buds. With all the shouting, I felt like I was back in Ikamatua.

'Ross is as exciting as its name': a description I had read. I actually found it to be charming. The Empire Hotel was certainly character-filled. I was still not drinking so just took a quick peek. There was a little shopfront around the corner, with motorcycle titbits sellotaped inside the window. Most of them were news clippings about speedway. Most people wouldn't even notice the store; it wasn't really a store – just a glass window and a door. Ross had several of these curiosities. Interesting nooks and crannies. It took a little time but there was character to be found in a place with such a bland name.

I was booked into the Ross Motels. I had booked as it was the only motel in town, and I didn't want to miss out. I needn't have bothered as I was the only guest.

There was the Top 10 Holiday Park by the beach, which offered boutique accommodation in converted shipping containers. It was $140 a night – bit steep for me. Also, I could sleep in a shipping container anytime I wanted.

The motel proprietor was lovely. She let me use her washing machine and drier for free. She showed me a shed where I could lock the bike. The motel was immaculate.

I decided to skip on a pub meal – to save money on food. What did the Four Square have on offer? Frozen packet lasagne and Chinese pork balls. I made the mistake of throwing away the packaging – it would have been tastier than the 'food'.

Ross to Fox

118km seal, 12km gravel

A cloud of ill disposition was about. I drew a curtain. It was an IPA sort of sky – not quite a hazy. I got listlessly into my tea and porridge – but food never tasted the same without a little love put into it – *don't throw your oats at the pot*; sprinkle them in it with care. I put a little extra honey in the tea – perhaps that would sweeten my temperament.

By now I could pack and dress while blindfolded – I even had the stocking fitting finessed. Loading the bike took only a few minutes. I bungeed the spare tyre on one bag and bungeed my jandals to the other, letting it go with a twang.

Ross to Hari Hari took me three hours. That was a 15kph average and included 12km of easy gravel – so, the pace was alright. It was the attitude.

The first couple of hours were usually hard work as I had to burn the remnants of the sleeping pill out of my system – the grogginess. Some would see that as a blessing, especially on a long, dull stretch of road when you didn't want an overactive brain.

I was an insomniac and as such was always in search of THE pill, the one that would give you a night's sleep and you would wake feeling sharp, full of beans. Not one that made your brain feel like a marmalade sponge. I was currently on Temazepam – recommended to be used only on rare occasions – not daily. I mused on the possibility that I could be addicted to it. *Yeah, nah.* It was giving me six hours sleep a night; I would take that. The first four hours were solid. The next two hours were assembled from the scatterings of sleep I cast about for in the craziness of the early hours. I had the most fantastic dreams during those periods; I just couldn't remember them. They could be exhausting, I knew, by the state I was in when I would finally awake. I could be in a sweat. Often, I would wake with bedding and clothes strewn about. If I was in my sleeping bag, the drawstring would be wrapped about my neck – that would be the S and M dreams.

I had tried Triazolam, Zopiclone, Nortriptyline, Serotonin, Melatonin and Amitriptyline. Codeine could work in the early hours, although it left you constipated. Valium was the best but you needed to know a doctor, (nudge, nudge, wink, wink). Morphine was heaven but you were usually in a place with lots of beeping and stethoscopes to get that – and there was the risk, that paradise could become the destination. Marijuana was probably the go, but I doubted whether I would have the will to get out of bed and cycle if I was toking up large in the night. I did know, on my return home, that there would be a reckoning with my doctor on the overuse of Temazepam.

(Ideally we would shoot a couple of snorts of ether and forget what the appointment was about.)

I was struggling with the doldrums. I was in a beautiful part of NZ, I had enough money for the trip, I didn't have to go to work, I was amongst spectacular mountains – but I couldn't actually see them because the cloud was low, in a drizzly wet kind of misty way. In fact, I hadn't seen any mountains since being on the west coast because of the low, drizzly, wet kind of cloud. And I wouldn't get to see any mountains until I climbed away from the west coast.

The attitude problem was possibly more to do with having been on the road on a cycle for long enough. Or was I just going through a lonely spell? Luigi collected wingmen, and wingwomen – perhaps that was a good idea? Perhaps that was what I needed. I had Homer – but let's face it: – Homer wasn't human.

I put on a podcast to keep my brain from wandering to bad places.

Hari Hari had a café – not much else, but I didn't need much else – besides something to adjust my mood.

The food selection contained some interesting choices. I went for the potato sausage roll. That's right – a sausage roll where the sausage had been replaced by potato. Perhaps they'd run out of sausage meat, I wondered, as I took the number the server gave me back to the table.

There were only three customers. I wasn't in a Ponsonby café bumping shoulders with a throng. You would think she could remember who I was without me needing a number. Besides, the other two customers had already been served. I was front running for the most cantankerous award this morning.

I glanced at the number, it was a 5. I had a small-minded game I played where I tried to match a number with the number that a motorcycle racer used. Valentino Rossi had the most famous number: 46. It could be found in the most unlikely places throughout the world. Number 5 was Colin Edwards, a legendary American rider. I had raced Edwards in Australia at the International Island Classic. Edwards was racing for the Yank team and I was in the Kiwi team. I had been part of the NZ team for several years and had had the chance to race many of the stars. Troy Corser, Jeremy McWilliams, John McGuinness, Peter Hickman, to name a few. To be honest, 'race', was a misuse of the word. I may have been in the same races, but I wasn't in the same contest. The guns, the stars, started at the front of the field and I started somewhere close to the back. I only got to see them at the start of the race and after it had finished. If I saw them during the race it would have been because I was being lapped; fortunately this didn't happen. The great novelty of the Island Classic was that amateurs, like me, got to race against professional racers. Even better was that we all mixed in together and it was a celebration of classic bikes and racing them. Park your ego at the door; no cocks allowed. Then there was number 5, Mr Edwards. He attended just the once. Colin had his own trailer he could retire to between races – so as not to be disturbed. I was not an unkind person – let's just say that I didn't think that Edwards had entered into the spirit of the meeting.

A couple of young lads pulled up outside the café, in an old Japanese car. On the roof was tied a young pig – a young dead pig. They had it tied from a leg at each end, down and through the windows. I would have felt embarrassed driving around with a pig tied on the roof – and one so small. I did not know the ways of these parts, however. It could have been part of some, becoming-a-man ritual.

Just south of Hari Hari was a 200-metre ridge called Mt Hercules. A big name for a little climb. I did appreciate that the coast was now putting some effort into its names. In fact, the west coast naming extravagance knew no bounds. After struggling to give away Westport, Blackball and Greymouth in the unimaginative names ballot, who wanted Ross? Just as well there were plenty of mothers about that thought it was a fine name.

The coast then went on something of a spree. It was as if the coast had gone on an OE and returned overflowing with ebullience. Hari Hari – 'Hare Rama, Rama Rama, Hari Krishna,' I chanted as I rode. I had hoped Hari Hari had its foundation in some far off, mystical land – such as that where Hare Krishna had its genesis; the USA. I couldn't have been further off-track. Hari Hari was Māori and meant, 'to carry joy' – kind of spiritual. However, Hari Hari had become Harihari in recent times, and not officially. Harihari meant ambulance in Māori.

Fox – NZ didn't even have foxes. But there were many just outside London, not far from Earl's Court. The origins of the names weren't nearly as exciting as I hoped. Fox was named after Sir William Fox, the second Premier of NZ. Fox headed NZ governments four times and was described as being a 'rug-puller' rather than a bridge-builder – he seemed happier when in opposition. I beat about in my political memory box for a modern-day equivalent: Winston Peters?

Then there was Mt Hercules – I could find no history of it, but I celebrated it anyway by chasing a white Volvo SUV down its slopes. The driver was clearly distressed by the mad cyclist up his chuff. His cornering lines went to pieces as he threw the car side to side in an effort to find more speed – unpleasant for his passenger. I felt a bit better about the world after that.

West Coast rivers changed course as often as Liz Taylor changed husbands. Their propensity to flood and drag large volumes of debris downstream could play havoc with Highway 6 – hence why many of the bridges appeared newish. The Waitangitaona River used to flow north to join the Whataroa River. In 1986 it had a change of plan and set out for Lake Wahapo and thence into the Ōkārito Lagoon. This change of course converted Lake Wahapo into a turbid body of water, killed a stand of Kahikatea trees and endangered SH6. Geographical cavalcades were about but I wasn't picking up the signs. I rode past the signpost for Ōkārito, it had been home for Keri Hulme for many years and there was a huge lagoon (NZ's largest natural wetland). I acknowledged that I must come back and put some time into the coast – but not on this trip.

The low cloud took away the vistas of snowclad peaks. Mizzle settled on me like Granny's moth-eaten blanket. My front wheel, on the wet tar, shot a jet of water up my crotch. All in all, it was a forgettable day.

Franz Josef had a smattering of tourists but the coast was doing it hard since Covid-19 had spoiled the party. The helicopters weren't flying because of the cloud.

I decided to put it in and get over the three peaks between Franz Josef and Fox, none of which had names despite being much taller than Mt Hercules. It was a 20km stretch. Put in the effort and save myself from having to do it in the morning. Plus, I had booked a motel in Fox.

It was another immaculate motel and another $100 for the night. But there was no way that I was going to stay in a wet and cold tent at this stage of the trip. Basic luxury was needed. I appeared again to be the only patron of the motel; tourism was in the doldrums.

Betsey Jane's was the place I went for dinner. I didn't personally know Betsey Jane – it was the name of the restaurant. It was also the closest restaurant to the motel. I was pleasantly surprised to find the place busy.

I ordered the lasagne but was told it was – you guessed it – not currently available. Still, I ate a fine meal of cod, chips and salad. I sat by myself in my jandals, shorts (with no underwear), my one clean shirt, and my puffer jacket.

Fox to Haast

122km seal

A morning malaise again hovered over me – just above pillow height. I lay perfectly still, on my back. Indisposition hung like a low, dark cloud. I tried to rationalise this feeling. 'In dis position I'm not going anywhere,' I breathed. 'Come on solider, get up, get moving.'

I was pretty sure it wasn't anything to do with being solo – that was my go-to setting. I had been in no mood to joke with Homer for the past couple of days. I was pretty sure it was to do with being back cycling on a main highway. It was a very quiet highway – but it was still a highway. Highway 6 to be precise. *That would make it 5 highways down from the absolute terror of Highway 1, right?*

A positive to take was that there was little cell phone coverage on the coast, so the likelihood of there being a texting youth behind the wheel was diminished. But still, the next car could be the last. *Please let it be a Chev.* But this was no joking matter. There was no shoulder on Highway 6. I had been told that South Island drivers were more considerate of cyclists than North Islanders. *Everyone was better than Northlanders.* I hadn't found South Islanders to be more considerate drivers, there were just less of them. I still tensed up on hearing a vehicle roaring up from behind. Could this be the one? The cold steel roar that was going to take me out – the last sound I would hear. Since 2017 there had been 24 cyclists killed on NZ roads.

'The highways are crowded with people who drive as if their sole purpose in getting behind the wheel is to avenge every wrong done them by man, beast or fate'. HST.

The Road Code stated that a minimum gap of 1.5 metres should be given to cyclists. The standard practice that I had observed in the past in my unofficial survey was for Kiwi motorists to put their outside wheel on, or just over, the centreline when passing a cyclist. That had changed. Kiwi motorists now attempted to pass cyclists within the *same* lane. And on open roads. *Why should they have to move over for some dickhead on a bike?* And whatever you do, don't slow down. Get past that cyclist as quickly as possible. Motorists saw cyclists as just another piece of 'road furniture' as they called it at the Isle of Man TT.

'Righteo, what's for breakfast?' I asked, to no-one in particular.

'Mmmmn beer. Get me a Duff.' Homer was awake. I took the bike inside at every chance – to keep it dry – and safe from theft; Homer benefitted.

'Surprise, surprise,' I said. 'It's tea and porridge.'

'Oh well,' said Homer.

It was a cold morning. I went for my usual attire of late: leg warmers, two pairs of chamois shorts, camo shorts, Glassons merino top, light waterproof/windbreaker, neck buff, skull cap and gloves. It was still that fine balance of keeping the chill off while not sweating too much. I would have preferred 30 degrees – but that wasn't happening anytime soon.

I got my head down and into my work down Highway 6; the legs were automatons. I crossed the Fox River, the Weheka River and the Ohinetamatea River. They were soon followed by the Karangarua River, the Manakaiaua River and Jacobs River – not to be mistaken for Jacobs Creek. There were about 50 single-lane bridges on the West Coast; no one could keep count – or keep up – because of the constant backtracking, backpedalling and reconsidering that were the nature of the rivers thereabouts. I hoped to meet an oncoming car on one of the bridges; the one where I had the right of way. Despite there being an abundance of abutments, I never encountered any cars on the bridges. I was very glad for the bridges – otherwise I would have gotten very wet.

The South Island was known for its lakes and rivers – not so much its beaches. (Now, there was an argument starter.) For a Northlander, like me, beaches had to reach a high benchmark to be called good. However, I rounded a bend and there was a picture-perfect beach. Bruce Bay was a lovely beach. Not, in a throw your clothes off and dash madly in, kind of way; it would have been freezing. But it was a very pleasant horseshoe shaped bay with sand and waves. Many West Coast beaches were steep-faced and downright dangerous for swimming. A persistent southwest swell, driven by the Roaring Forties, drove sand and gravel up the shores. Bruce Bay was a small patch of calm.

I was into the last section of coastline before turning inland. My next glimpse of sea would be on the run into Bluff.

I went again to some podcasts for comfort. The one I had selected for the morning was called, 'Going the Wrong Way,' by Chris Donaldson. Donaldson, a young man in the early 70's, left his hometown of Belfast to ride a café-style MotoGuzzi to Australia. For the uneducated, a café-style motorcycle was not one with a parasol on the back, under which was placed a cappuccino on a chequered tablecloth. It was a sporty style of bike most suited to fast, curvy sealed roads.

Donaldson had more than his share of adventures as many of the places he went had no roads. He wasn't so much off the beaten track, he was beating the track.

Donaldson had had to eat some extremely dodgy meals. I had done the same in my time and I was now about to go, eyes wide open, back to a venue where bad things had previously happened. I had mostly good experiences with food on this trip. The biggest difficulty, especially in Northland, had been finding food – finding a place that was open.

It was 120km from Fox to Haast and the Salmon Farm Café at Paringa stood exactly in the middle. A cyclist needed fuel to keep going – that captive market thing again.

I had been to the Salmon Farm a few months earlier while holidaying in the South Island. The farm featured four large circular pools with salmon at different stages of life swimming about in them.

You could look down on the pools from a balcony. The balcony was next to the café.

Against my better judgement, and to my wife's amusement, I had ordered salmon fillets. I wasn't a big fan of salmon. But if it was cooked right, like you would a steak, it could be alright. I reasoned that if you were going to eat salmon, then eat if fresh. Go to the source. My wife smiled; she'd been here before. Not the salmon farm, but with me in this situation. I liked to try things – new experiences. To see if there were adventures to be had in food. Usually there were. Sometimes they were good.

So long as they cooked the salmon, *just so*. I couldn't abide the thought of it being soft and squishy.

'I'll have the salmon fillets. Can you cook them crispy?' I asked cheerfully, of the large lady behind the counter. They were all large attendants in the kitchen. I took this as a good sign. Usually meant they liked their food and knew how to cook. Well, fry, at least.

'You mean battered?' asked the lady.

'No,' I said, softly. *How could I explain this?* 'I want to be able to taste the salmon. But can you cook them dry?'

She arched an eyebrow and looked closely at me. To see if I was taking the piss. 'So, you want them deep fried.'

'Not exactly,' I said, frowning. Searching for the explanation that wasn't coming. 'Just not soggy. Like, drier fillets. Not wet ones.'

Well, I completely fucked that, I thought, as we seated ourselves at a table from which we could see the farm salmon swimming in mindless circles.

I was doomed. My wife had begun laughing lightly as I dug and dug my hole. Once the hole was deep enough, you could stop digging. But oh no, I was determined to dig that sucker deeper and deeper.

One of the kitchen hands had disappeared downstairs, soon after I put my order in. No doubt to dispatch a salmon and clean the guts out. She reappeared with a small Tupperware box.

The salmon was delivered to me on a bed of languid lettuce. Two pale fillets lying bland and limp. I gave my wife a despairing look, dropped my brow and raised the knife and fork.

'It's probably the healthiest thing I'll eat for a while,' I mumbled, as I forced a forkful down. The last mouthful didn't want to go down and I had to push the fork into my mouth twice to get the fish down.

The waitress had forgotten the poached egg; so had I. It was a part of the meal. It arrived late, by itself, wobbling in a small bowl. I nearly retched – I stole away to the bathroom.

I could have sworn that an hour later the fillets reformed in my stomach into a ghost salmon, that began slowly swimming laps. Round and round in my gut as we drove the hills of the west coast. I had gone for a milkshake in Haast in the misbegotten belief that milk would soothe my stomach. Kill the ghost salmon – *seriously?* Fortunately for me, they were out of cups and so couldn't do milkshakes. I went instead for deep fried cod and chips – by now my culinary instincts had totally abandoned me. I also bought a box of tea bags and some milk.

The afternoon ended up with us parked in our campervan and the kettle on. A nice cup of tea to wash the awful nightmare away. Dulp, I had bought Earl Grey teabags by mistake.

On this visit, I ordered a bagel and a chocolate muffin; stay safe. They didn't do milkshakes, so I got a smoothie. Surely, they could do a half-decent job of serving that up.

And that's exactly what they did: A half-decent job. The bagel was as limp as the salmon fillets I had on the last trip there. The muffin looked a million dollars; it was a trap. Chocolate icing was lavished on it, and it was sticky. Sticky like that saying about stuff sticking to a blanket. So sticky that it got on my fingers and wouldn't come off. Even stickier than butt cream. Viscous and clinging. I tried licking it, but it had the consistency of tar. The icing preferred to stay on my fingers. The thin napkin was a waste of time – it just tore and got stuck in clumps on the end of my fingers.

I went to the bathroom, using my elbows to open the doors, and washed my hands clean. I then returned to the table. If my wife had been there, well, I knew that this experience would have become a family heirloom.

Is there a camera somewhere? I wondered. Am I being set up, like on Candid Camera? ('Oh, he's come back. Here he comes now. Get out the sticky icing, this should be fun.')

The thing was, the place was busy. Being 50 or 60 kilometres from the next town meant you could expect tourists to stop to dine. I revolved in my seat to regard my fellow diners. They were mostly older, as was the norm for this time of year. They appeared to be having a good time. No one was putting on a horror show — lifting their hands to display a ghastly web of chocolate icing.

Best I left. Move on. Get out of that place and never darken its doorway again.

The scenery was lovely down this part of the coast and culminated at the Knights Point lookout, a popular stopping point for tourists. A great place for a café, I thought, bitterly. *Move on, son.*

She could be rugged out in those waters, the Tasman Sea. I observed a couple of runabouts fishing off a point. Good to boat in pairs. In case one gets in trouble. Open ocean there. Next stop, Tasmania.

A few tourists noticed my bicycle and all the claptrap attached to it — took a little interest in it. A couple of them nodded to me, one gave a thumbs up. A middle-aged man wanted to know where I had come from and where I was going. People's eyes would often go wide when I told them.

'Hey, hon,' he called, to his wife. 'Come and look at this. This fella has biked down from North Cape and is going to The Bluff.'

'Cape Reinga, actually,' I said. I couldn't help myself. People often said North Cape, mistaking it for Cape Reinga. And I wasn't going to The Bluff. It was just, Bluff.

'Oh, look at you,' said the man's wife. 'Riding all these hills must be exhausting.'

'I'm used to it by now,' I smiled. 'I actually like the hills. Find them more interesting.'

'How are you finding all the cars?' she asked. 'Kiwis are pretty good on the whole around bikes.'

I paused. She had framed the question in a way that wanted confirmation. She had gone for the 'new' style of journalism. Make a statement and wait for the interviewee to validate the statement. Paint a picture, put it in a statement and launch it on the interviewee: even if you've just said that, because your father kept goats, he had a thing for goats. When did asking a question stop being the normal term of engagement for a journalist? This bubbly and seemingly lovely woman wanted confirmation that Kiwis were good motorists and considerate of cyclists. *Why not just sell your soul.*

'No,' I said. 'Kiwis are the worst drivers in the world, I think. They are awful around cyclists. So help them if they had to take their foot off the gas for just a few seconds.'

'Oh,' she said. This rude biker wasn't following the rules of etiquette. 'Well, have a nice ride.' The couple hurried away to find another lookout.

Was that necessary? Should I be taking out my Salmon Farm chocolate muffin experience on that poor woman?

It was dangerous riding a motorcycle on NZ roads with all the subtle traps laid to catch the unwary; or unlucky rider. Gravel thinly veiled on a corner. Diesel splashes on asphalt, especially after rain. Gape-mouthed potholes. Off-camber bitumen rolled into a nasty wrinkle by heavy trucks. All sorts of snares to take a biker down. Add to that the Kiwi motorist who transformed into an obstinate, demonic, nasty piece of work behind the wheel and it was a miracle a motorcyclist could even pull the bed covers down past his chin come the morning. The French had a saying: **rouler à tombeau ouvert**.

It meant driving with your coffin open – a debonair way to describe a motorcyclist. New Zealanders often called riders 'temporary kiwis.'

Cycling was an even more dangerous habit than motorcycling; you had no power to escape; you were in effect a large possum in the headlights.

Haast was to be my last port of call on the coast. I didn't want to admit it, but I was glad. It had been good cycling weather – cool and no wind. Only occasional light rain – nothing like the rain the coast was notorious for. The accommodation had been, without fail, superb.

I just felt like I was marking time rather than making time. The k's had been good but it felt a little endless. Once over Haast Pass, I felt sure it would be all downhill from there.

Roadkill was much in evidence on the coast. I was used to the possum carnage up north, with the occasional pukeko thrown in. But traffic was light on the coast, yet the possum kill was high. I couldn't help noticing the lushness of the possum fur down south. In Northland the possums were a motley grey colour and the coat was short. Down south the possums had thick, rich pelts. Chocolate brown, *like muffin icing.*

There was time to observe the possums in all their gory – one advantage of travelling slowly by bicycle. Their coats were luxuriant and they appeared to be very healthy – well, not that healthy – they were dead.

Was it a cheap thrill a possum was after in that madcap loitering about on the road in front of the headlights? Or some form of initiation? Bildungsroman for possum? The ultimate kudos: to be able to hang out there in all that blinding white light until the very last moment before skittering off the road, narrowly avoiding the squashing impact of the black radials. It called for split-second timing to get it right. A possum would have to build a fine sense of precognition to get it right. It wasn't the sort of activity one wanted to practice; it was a one chance grab. Or was it just blind luck that most possums got it right? Perhaps it was an endlessly dull life that drove them to take on the tar dance of death. 'What's for dinner?' 'Leaves.' 'What, again?'

Who really knew? But it was a kinky mess of craziness when 70 watts of halogen were bearing down on you. Why did the possum cross the road? To see his flatmate; my one bleak possum joke.

There wasn't much choice for accommodation in Haast; it was a rather austere place. It had a hunkered down for bad weather vibe – a little like National Park. A place you passed through, as if the people living there had stopped for gas and forgot to get going again.

Haast River Motels was to be the night's abode. The girl at reception was a little confused that I had arrived by bicycle. The booking form clearly had a slot for a registration number. She asked me innocently if I had a number plate. Cute.

Another cook in the bag meal. This time it was roast lamb. Unlike McDonalds food, each cook in the bag meal did taste different from the last – and you got plenty.

'Tomorrow we climb,' I said, to myself – and Homer. *Is that what Sir Ed would have said to Tenzing Norgay Sherpa?* I didn't have a Sherpa but I did have Homer. Homer got to sleep inside again. I only left the bike out when I was camping or there was no shed to lock it in. I got a towel and wiped the moisture off the bike. I gave Hal a rub down too – got rid of any rain and road grime.

'Mmmmn beer,' murmured Homer happily, as he drifted off.

Homer had been strangely quiet for the past few days – pretty much since he had broken his arm – or more correctly, as Homer liked to point out, since I had broken his arm.

Haast to Makarora

78km seal

It was another cool morning with low cloud obscuring the mountains. No breeze. Good weather for mountain climbing. Oatmeal, banana and a bit of honey – breakfast of champions.

I got away at daybreak, as was my wont – between 8 and 8.30. The morning was spent moving up a gentle incline through a pleasant river valley containing the Haast River (Māori called it Awarua). It wasn't always so calm: huge amounts of sediment were regularly moved from the Southern Alps to the sea. Headwards sapping occurred when the ridge between two rivers was devoured by the more vigorous river. This occurred right down the coast but was very evident on the Haast. The valley was the beginning of the Mt Aspiring National Park and was classified as a World Heritage site; it was certainly grand. The pass got its name from Julius von Haast who explored a route from Otago to the West Coast – a trail that was long known to Māori.

I pulled up at the 50km mark: Pleasant Flat Recreational Area. *Whoever named it that had a sense of humour.* The sandflies came in like Messerschmitts. I pulled the neck buff over my face. The buggers ransacked their way down my body sniffing for flesh – the ankle being the dream find. I got out of there in a hurry, no smoko that morning.

I pedalled a few corners, to get clear of the sandflies, and dismounted; it was time for a long walk – fine by me. Waterfalls cascaded off rock ledges to fall hundreds of metres to deep green pools. Mountains towered on both sides of the road – the pass was a deep cut in the landscape. The pace was slow but steady, I stopped often to take in a new marvel. The Roaring Billy Falls Walk. Thunder

Creek Falls Walk. Fantail Falls Walk. If you were into waterfalls then this was falls nirvana.

The road climbed 500 metres in only a few kilometres making this one of the steepest passes on the TA. There was no shoulder but very little traffic – I could hear any vehicles coming. Being so steep and a bit winding kept the speed of vehicles to a moderate level.

In 1900, a fellow by the name of AP Harper was the first person to bike and hike over Haast Pass. Imagine that? I couldn't.

There was no lookout or cairn to signify the top of Haast Pass. I suspected I had gone over it as the road slope changed, but you never could be sure – I'd been caught out before by false peaks. My speed increased and I found myself behind two beekeeping trucks. I could tell they were beekeeping trucks because they had hives on the back – and the hives appeared to be fully occupied.

The drivers were keeping their speed well down, so as to not lose any bees. I could have overtaken but didn't think this would be serendipitous. Besides, the trucks would eventually take me back again. And besides that, the smell was heaven.

Over the top of the pass and it felt as if the heavens had peeled back. The dark blanket of the west coast ended. Blue sky was ahead and warm sunlight filtered down on me. Then a tailwind sprang up – and not just any tailwind but a peal of air from an angel's mouth. I was cruising at nearly 30kph.

I whistled past the Blue Pools. The huge parking area was busy with campervans. A very popular stop but there was no stopping me this day – I was riding this zephyr. My destination was Makarora and the Wonderland Lodge. I had heard great things about it.

I arrived at Wonderland at 2pm. It was almost embarrassing how easy it had been with the tailwind. I felt as if I should keep going; cyclists didn't turn down tailwinds. However, the man in the office said it was the prevailing wind and it would be there the next day. I had a sandwich, and a milkshake – I chewed on whether to push on to my mate's at Wanaka – I was a traveller now, so I could stop without guilt. Wonderland featured cute A-framed lodges. Each one was set within its own copse of trees. At $70, I was pleased. It had all the mod cons. The bathroom was shared. I decided to stay the night.

There was a BBQ being put on for a corporate group that was holding a conference at Wonderland. This seemed a little incongruous – corporate, wonderland. Perhaps two words that had never been used in the same sentence.

I wasn't in the corporate mood and instead went for another cook in the bag dehydrated meal. Beef and pasta hotpot this time.

Makarora to Wanaka

54km seal, 20km cycle path

Needless to say, there was no tailwind for me that morning. There was no wind at all. I would take that and besides, it wasn't a long ride, it was a beautifully fine day and the scenery was going to be superb. Breakfast of champions and away by 8.30.

If you had to cycle on a main road, this was surely one to choose in NZ. It bordered Lake Wanaka on the left and climbed and bounded and rolled. There was no shoulder, which was a concern to me, as this was rubber necking country – drivers could be easily distracted by the vistas. Massive ledges pitched at crazy angles and soared into the heights – there had been some serious interglacial upheavals. Thor had been swinging his hammer.

There was a curious sign on the side of the road for the attention of cyclists. It was done in stick figure and pictured a cyclist pitching forward over the handlebars of his bike. The bike had no front wheel. I reckoned this was probably the reason for the cyclist pitching forward. The artist begged to differ and was instead indicating that there was a ditch or culvert in the road – so beware.

At the 25km mark I climbed up a section called The Neck. Lake Wanaka and Lake Hawea were created by the advances of great glaciers that carved out their bowls. The ice flows connected through this saddle. Emerald blue lakes on either side, sharp edged mountain peaks running away into the sky. It was beauty beyond man's ability, the work of the gods – too grand for words.

The road switched lakes at The Neck, running down to the town of Hawea.

I rang my mate, Simon, who lived in Wanaka. Simon kindly offered to bring his van to pick me up – to save me having to cycle the 25km to Wanaka. Imagine that. *Who would know I'd caught a lift? Cheated. I would. Bloody hell.*

Hawea was still a one store town – I didn't think it had changed much in the past 40 years. A groomed cycle trail began just down from the shop. It initially ran beside a manmade stream with crystal clear water from Lake Hawea – going somewhere. I didn't want to strain my brain working out where it was going; it was just nice that it was going. There was a manmade wave built in the Hawea River. I stopped to watch a kayaker playing up and down the face of it – other kayakers awaited their turn. I wondered how the wave was made. Then my brain really did hurt.

A cool swing bridge took the trail over Hawea River. Hawea River then roared away to join the Clutha River on a ride to Lake Dunstan. Lake Dunstan was manmade – like the wave. There was controversy when the lake was made. The original Cromwell was now at the bottom of the lake. The residents had to upsticks and move to the site where a new Cromwell township was being built. A booze up was had in the old hotel on the eve of the flooding of the lake. I bet the publican checked to make sure his watch hadn't stopped.

Wanaka was a boomtown. There was no other way to describe it. Subdivisions and clusters of houses were growing faster than cancer. One bonus of Covid-19 shutting down the tourist trade was that Wanaka residents were now able to go to town – were now able to get to town without needing to take leave to wait in the queue. It was much more civilized.

Small town NZ was growing rapidly; I had noticed this on the trip. Most town authorities embraced the extra revenue provided by immigrants; most residents complained about the lack of parking spaces and the crowds. Crowds was a relative term: A New York crowd at the traffic lights was different to a Te Kuiti crowd at the traffic lights.

Simon lived in a new subdivision with splendid views away to the mountains. He collected classic rally cars. He liked to drive fast, and he didn't appreciate cyclists blocking up the roads. His view was that they should make themselves scarce when he was about. Keep hard left – God help you if you were two abreast.

'This is the fast lane, folks…and some of us like it here.'
—*HST*

Wanaka to Queenstown

45km seal, 3km gravel, 37km cycle trail

The classic Cardrona Hotel stood on the lower slopes of the Crown Range. It drew you in. The old wooden hotel with an ancient Chrysler car rusting outside. Established in 1863, the hotel was one of NZ's oldest and one of only two remaining buildings from the Cardrona Valley gold rush era. I wasn't drawn in for long though, as there was no cabinet food to be had in the hotel. Instead, I went across the road to the Cardrona Valley General Store where a full cabinet of delectables awaited. Brilliant, and they served milkshakes. I did a quick Google search on the general store – not much info available. A reviewer had put that there was nothing there for vegetarians. I guessed the interpretation of vegetarian must have changed. I didn't know cheese scones and blueberry muffins were now persona non grata for vego's. Hard to keep up.

I had been eating pretty healthily, all in all, on the trip. After the initial hiccups with carb loading, I had gone the protein way if possible during the day – and it had worked. In truth, I was probably eating no more than I did when I was at home. Except, of course, for the milkshakes – I wasn't bombing one or two milkshakes a day at home.

I was as confused as anybody by the new fads on eating. Being vegetarian was radical back in the day. I had a friend who had tried going fruitarian. That didn't work well unless one wanted to spend a lot of time on the toilet and dramatically lose weight. Probably a good diet if you were going travelling in India – to prepare yourself. Then there was the pescatarian. Or the vegan, that looked like a tough row to hoe.

The good news was that nowadays you could really eat or drink anything you wanted and it was going to be kosher in some category. I leaned towards the 'eat anything that has a parent' category. Lettuces were people too.

The Crown Range road had no shoulder. Like the Haast Pass, there were a lot of metal cages and nets at the sides to catch falling rocks. There were also a lot of Armco barriers, so it was hard to get over to the far left when cars came from behind – Simon wasn't on the road that morning. The last few kilometres were tough as the road steepened noticeably.

I had forsworn podcasts in favour of talking books. I had a couple downloaded on my phone. The one I chose for the Crown Range climb was *Jaws* – the novel by Peter Benchley written in 1974. The movie that kept Kiwis out of the water for the summer. The talking book didn't have the pounding music when the shark was attacking. That was a shame, I reckoned. Could be motivational music for hills.

It was 40 kilometres of climbing – 500 metres within 12kms at its steepest to reach the summit at 1100 metres.

Campervans and cars were parked in the large carpark. You could see all the way down to Lake Wakatipu – it was a peach of a day. Bright sunlight and a few puffy clouds to complement the picture. I dug out an apple and enjoyed the view, however, I didn't linger as the wind was cold. Going downhill on a bicycle could be quicker than taking a car – it was all to do with physics: rolling mass to be exact. I easily caught a large Maui campervan. I passed it, giving a wave while still munching away on the apple. *Show off.*

This is too much fun, I thought, throwing the core over the guardrail. A chance for a little payback where the bike was mightier than the car.

I had to work hard to get up behind the next vehicle. Frantic pedalling in top gear soon put me behind a Toyota Highlander. I took it on the outside of a bend, which surprised both myself and the driver.

There were no other vehicles in sight, besides which, I had to veer off the Crown Range Road onto Glencoe Road, a gravel road that led towards Arrowtown. Then it was down Tobins Track, a 4WD path that dropped dramatically into Arrowtown.

Arrowtown was its usual lovely self and busy with tourists – nowhere near as busy as it was before the pandemic, but still bustling.

The Queenstown Trail was the picture-perfect path in the album of perfect cycle trails. Stunning scenery and smooth road-like tracks took me from Arrowtown to Queenstown via five bridges, all of them very cool. I was staying at my daughter's in Lower Shotover. Lower Shotover conjured up greater visions than Lower Hutt. (At the crack of dawn I would be fired out of a cannon over the water – as opposed to being sent from the Hutt.)

However, I had to make the dawn. I got struck by a migraine a couple of k's from Lower Shotover. I figured it was all the bright sunlight that caused it. I had been without sun on the West Coast and now it was all a bit much. Flickering vision began in my left eye and pretty soon took over the whole landscape. I swallowed some aspirin that I carried in case of such situations. It didn't stop the migraine but helped the recovery – maybe – it was a theory.

My vision went so haywire that I appeared to be riding in a blizzard – a crazed kaleidoscope of shattered visual fragments. If I used the peripheral vision in my right eye, I could just discern a distorted cycleway. My speed dropped to single digits.

I felt like Scott in a snowstorm trying to reach the South Pole – a 25-degree Celsius snowstorm. It was a nightmare trying to find the house. Lower Shotover was a new subdivision and all the houses wore a common theme – black corrugated iron and cedar panels. Flat roofs.

My daughter's partner, Jake, was building a storage shed out the front of their place. The storage shed defined the house from the others. This was the object I was navigating to, left eye blind and right eye squinted closed.

I found the house, found the key under the pot plant, and collapsed on the couch.

'Haaaayyy, wassup!,' greeted Jake, when he arrived home.

I peeked at him sideways. Partly because he was my daughter's boyfriend, but mostly because that was the only way of seeing him. My eyesight was slowly returning.

Queenstown to Mossburn

Boat trip, 103km gravel and cycle trail

I actually had to leave before the crack of dawn as I was catching a water taxi from downtown QT at 9am. So, it was a sprint in the dark with no lights.

> Hello darkness, my old friend
> I've come to talk with you again
> Because a vision softly creeping
> Left its seeds while I was sleeping
> And the vision that was planted in my brain
> Still remains
> Within the sound of silence
>
> In restless dreams I walked alone
> Narrow streets of cobblestone
> 'Neath the halo of a street lamp
> I turned my collar to the cold and damp
> When my eyes were stabbed by the flash of a neon light
> That split the night
> And touched the sound of silence

The boat wasn't there when I arrived. This did make me a bit panicky as I thought I'd missed it. The crew of another boat reassured me that it was still coming, I was fine. Relax.

The official guide said that QT was the 'busiest and most expensive tourist town in NZ'. Had the author visited Matamata? I had time to buy a massive bean burrito for $8 and a coffee for $4. Even sheep-shagging towns in the middle of the country were more expensive than that. QT had it all in spades and its network of MTB trails was world class. There was a reason the Twenty-Somethings naturally drifted there.

The water taxi duly arrived at the wharf. The skipper was so laid back he was practically asleep. Covid-19 had killed the international tourist trade but he was still running the routes despite the downturn.

NZ was the envy of the world with it being free of Covid-19 but freedom could be a fickle thing. The rest of the world had given up trying to eradicate the virus and were full tilt in trying to vaccinate against it. New Zealanders were dragging on getting the needle. 'She'll be right, mate, no Covid in God's own.'

Many people were nervous about getting a vaccine which had only recently been invented. Then there were the anti-vaxxers. In my lifetime there had been jabs for meningitis A and B, hepatitis A and B, typhoid, tetanus, polio, rabies, malaria, polio, rubella, mumps, whooping cough and diphtheria.

I was the only passenger. I felt pretty special, and a little guilty – a whole boat laid on just for me and my bike. Lake Wakatipu was calm and the taxi knifed a line straight through it to Walter Peak Station. The station was a popular tourist trap usually but of course with Covid all was silent as I pedalled by.

The first section of gravel road hugged the shore of Lake Wakatipu. Up the valley, far, far away was Mt Cook. *Was that really Mt Cook?* I was confused. My geography was up the *crapadoodle*. It was more likely Mt Aspiring, but …

A tailwind sprang up 10km out of Walter Peak Station – where the road turned left at Mt Nicholas Station. Shortly after this I came across an elderly couple on e-bikes – they had stopped for a sandwich. I was pleased they had e-bikes as they had a strong headwind to battle into – the wind was forecast to get even stronger.

Further along were four younger people pressing into the steady breeze. They appeared fresh as daisies and looked like they had just stepped out of a Kathmandu brochure. Their condition was astounding considering they were punting into a building headwind. Hadn't they just come over the 300-metre Von Hill? They too were on e-bikes. *Something fishy here*, I thought. They didn't look like cyclists – their cadence was too high for a start. Still, they were having a great time.

It wasn't until I rounded the next bend that it became clear. There was a van with a trailer at the base of Von Hill. The trailer had bike racks. The driver had just dropped the cyclists and was now packing up to drive around to QT to meet them. They got to ride through beautiful scenery to Lake Wakatipu. At Walter Peak Station the Earnslaw would arrive to ferry them back to QT in style. Nice. Very nice. Well done, those people.

Meanwhile, I ground my way up Von Hill. It wasn't a particularly tough climb and at this stage of the tour, no problem; it could even be called enjoyable. From Von Hill the scenery grew vast, the landscape cleaved open. A serious valley lay before me. Sweeping mountains rose on both sides, climbing to craggy peaks. It was like something from Jurassic Park. I half-expected stegosaurus and woolly mammoth to be grazing. I had never been in scenery like this – perhaps some parts of the Scottish Highlands were similar. I was blown away – both figuratively and literally as the wind had now increased dramatically.

Von Lake was nearby. It was only accessible with the landowner's permission. What made it phenomenal was that it was landlocked and yet had a strong population of rainbow trout. The trout had developed a method of spawning that allowed them to flourish. There were reportedly some big suckers in the lake.

I could pedal in top gear with little effort. This was fast – and a little too fast. The bike took on an uncanny weave. I had a fair idea about what could happen next. It involved the front wheel sliding into a gravel rut and then bad tumbling.

'Hey, whoa pal,' barked Homer. 'We're out of control.' The

combination of speed and corrugated gravel travelled a harsh vibration from the wheel, up the forks, up the head tube to the steering stem, to Homer; his feet screwed tight.

I backed it off one sprocket and the bike settled into a happy place. 'Sorry about that, little matey. She nearly got away on me.'

'Yeah, well keep it down a bit, pal. Some of us are trying to sleep.'

The pace was extraordinary with the strong Northerly. The mountains on either side regretfully subsided to become hills – but huge ones. A signpost read Mavora Lakes. Now, those were worth a visit. Imaginatively called the North and South lakes. Part of the Lord of the Rings trilogy was filmed there; it was that kind of scenery.

At one point there was a road with a sign for Te Anau. It was only 45km away. Incredible; I felt a little lost. It was such different terrain to anything I had ever experienced in NZ. Big sky country in a small country.

The valley then opened out to pasture. The gravel road continued, straight and long. I was glad for the tailwind as it was a fair haul to Mossburn. The graphs in the guide indicated it was pretty much all downhill from there to Bluff. I'd been told often that going from the top of NZ to the bottom was the trick, as it was downhill. I hadn't quite believed this – but, maybe there was something to it after all. I was also told once that the rivers in NZ flowed to the North – the country was basically upside down.

I wasn't worried. What was concerning me was the action playing out in my ear buds. They needed to clear the beaches in Amity asap as the shark was well into its bloody work. Matt Hooper, the hot biologist, had just arrived in Amity to give his version on what type of shark this was. Police chief Brody's wife was already eyeing Hooper up as a nice distraction from her mundane life.

A young woman was ahead, walking the gravel in the same direction as me. I pulled up beside her. She was walking the Te Araroa Trail and had emerged from a mountain track just a few kilometres back. She too, finished her trip at Bluff. The end was in sight but first she had to walk these long, long stretches of gravel. I, for the second time that day, felt a little guilty at the advantage I had. The walker didn't seem fazed – she had a stoic self-assurance about her that was admirable. The Tour Aotearoa was hard but the Te Araroa was *proper* hard – that was in a whole different league. It too was 3000 km long but followed a different course. Te Araroa meant, 'The Long Path'. I had mis-read it, at first, as 'The Long Pain'. At an average of 25kms a day, it took 120 days. The fastest known time for the Te Araroa was 49 days. The fastest time for the TA was eight days. The Te Araroa had long stretches away from civilisation – also known as shops. Hikers became very hungry and had hellacious visions of burgers, ice-creams, fish and chips, lollies and beer. TA'ers had none of that to deal with – there was always going to be a shop. However, I had enough on my nightmare plate, with Jaws to deal with.

I was glad to reach Mossburn – I was tired. That bone weary feeling. The penultimate day and I was ready for the end. The Mossburn Railway Hotel was the place for the last night before the end of the TA – another classic NZ hotel. The staff were super friendly and walked me through the warren of halls, showing me the kitchen, the bathrooms, the shed for the bike and my room.

The good staff of the hotel were used to dealing with travellers who'd been on the road for a good long while – whether walkers or bikers or explorers. The manager informed me that the walkers and cyclists were a real bonus – especially in March when the bulk of the TA'ers passed through. I didn't recall having been to Mossburn before – it was another blink and you'll miss it place. A couple of older fellas were sitting outside at a picnic table near the back door, near my room. They were removing their boots and woolly socks, which were a little damp. They had been fishing the Oreti River that day. I hadn't even realised that the gravel route had been following the Oreti River; I had been a little disorientated. The river flowed from the Mavora Lakes and it was known as a world class trout river. *Well, I never.*

A couple of even older fellas were in the carpark. They both had dogs in boxes on the back of their flatdecks – Toyota's of course. They were dog trialists. They were in Mossburn to compete in the nationals. I thought it was great that they were keeping the dying sport alive. Sports throughout NZ were dying, and it was only good, keen men such as these that were breathing life into them.

Steady on, hold your horses. The men enthusiastically informed me that dog trialing was very much alive and there were plenty of young people competing. I was chuffed to hear that dogs were being trialed throughout NZ in a sport with new life – just don't let them swim at Amity Beach.

One of the trialists favoured the short head and yard event. The other was more into the zig zag hunt. Neither of them was much interested in the long head or straight run. I felt that I now had enough information. I was pleased the sport was in good health and on the up – however, I could sense that the men thought that they had rounded up a captive ear, a chance for them to imbibe the nuances of dog trialling. Pretty soon they would have me scooting around the yard on all fours, tail wagging madly, sitting on command and going to fetch.

Leave it, Ben.

I got off all fours and made a break for my room

The last supper was held in the high studded dining room adjacent to the public bar. The bar looked to be doing a good trade. It gave me a warm feeling to know that in the far corners of NZ, people were still out there doing it despite the gravity of the Covid-19 situation.

I had the fettucine. There was plenty of it, enough to feed a small Italian family. I had wanted the lasagne, of course, but they had stopped cooking it the month before; they had forgotten to take it off the menu.

The waitress was a great salesperson. I observed her trying to push the gooseberry shortcake on the other patrons. It was either terrific shortcake, or awful, and they wanted to get shot of it. I was sure it was the former but the problem was that the mains were so large, everyone was full. I really wanted some but there was no way. In hindsight I should have taken a piece for the morrow.

Mossburn to Bluff

97km seal, 44km gravel

It was the last day of the TA. High cloud greeted me as I pulled back the curtains. The forecast was for rain, more so, later in the day – a time to pull out the oilskin if you were working your dogs.

Two elderly women were in the kitchen making sandwiches. They were the wives of the two dog handlers. No, shepherds, was the correct term, I corrected myself. Or, was shepherds an after-match term? During the event they would be dog trialists? It was a bit much to sort at that hour of the morning. They did have to be a member of the NZ Sheep Dog Trial Association (NZSDTA). That was up there for up there for one of the longest acronyms. I belonged to the NZ Classic Motorcycle Race Register (NZCMRR). That was pretty long.

They hadn't taken sandwiches for the trials, the day before. That had been a mistake as the food was expensive – $15 for a hamburger. Fine if you were one of the front runners as dog trialling paid big prize money.

The shepherds were out the back of the hotel giving their dogs a run-around before the day kicked off. I waited a spell before retrieving my bike from the shed – I didn't want to find myself again in the carpark rounding up imaginary sheep. I waited until the shepherds had gone inside to Tux into their breakfast.

Breakfast was included in the price. It was the last day and I forsook the breakfast of champions. I went instead for Weet-Bix and toast with marmalade – live a little dangerously.

Jaws was in the earbuds first thing – if a dose of terror and some exercise didn't clear the fog of a sleeping pill, what would?

Hooper, the biologist, was now into a mating ritual with chief Brody's wife, Ellen. The talking book went to some lengths to point out how great Ellen's body was even after having children. I thought that the author probably had some mother/son personal issues he was using the book to try to work through. The movie hadn't gone into any relationship between Hooper and Ellen. It was definitely a major part of the talking book and got pretty saucy.

'While shepherds wash their socks by night,' I sang, as I rode.

The gravel road gave way to board walk and cycle track through an area known as the Castle Downs Swamp. A lot of work had been put in to build this section – it was very cool. This was part of the Around the Mountains Cycle Trail that was extremely popular. Tour companies offered all sorts of packages – there was a trail ride suited to all levels of age and fitness. You could ride the whole thing and get your bags transported. You could ride a part, or parts of it. You could stay in the shuttle van the whole way if you wanted – watch your cycling mates from behind the windscreen. Smart tourism. I was a benefactor of it as the trail was very well kept.

There was pretty much no traffic for the first few hours; it was a Saturday. I decided to keep a log in my head of the traffic. Eight cars passed me in the first three hours and one truck. The truck and trailer unit was carrying bulk fertiliser. It was a long open road with no traffic. The driver decided to give me the good old brushback and get as close as he could.

The last day of the tour and this arsehole puts the full stop on all that I hated about being on the open road with Kiwi drivers. But come on mate, don't let this prick put a dampener on the last day of the TA. Besides, I had bigger fish to fry. Namely Jaws.

Chief Brody, Hooper (the biologist who was shagging Brody's wife), and the skipper of the charter boat, Quint, were now beginning an intimate relationship with the big fish. Quint and Jaws appeared to have taken an instant dislike to each other. I knew that this didn't end well for Quint. But that was the film, this was the book.

It was easy running into Winton. I stopped for an omelette and a milkshake. Would be rude not to, being the last day. A nondescript café on a grey day. Winton was only 30km from Invercargill. It was named after a farmer – hardly riveting. It could have been named instead after Minnie Dean. She was the only woman to be hanged in NZ; she was buried in the Winton Cemetery. Minnie took in unwanted children, no questions asked. A couple of them perished in her care. Dodgy dealings? – or, perhaps she just got a bad rap.

There were more exciting naming possibilities for the town. It could do with a bit of sparkle. Hangman's Noose. Minnie's Demise. Minnieville.

I also stopped at Wallacetown – a town with a population of 400 people. Murphy's Dairy and Takeaways was the happening place. There were a lot of utes in the carpark. The drivers of the pickups all looked to be cut from the same mould – gumboots, stubbies, fluro workshirts and hair cut as close to a mullet as was possible.

They all looked likely to be called Wallace – or perhaps, Murphy. I went for a piece of cod to celebrate the local fishery – and a vanilla milkshake.

The Invercargill cycle trail began just before the city. I picked it up off Dee St – it skirted the city and ran parallel with Bill Richardson Drive. Bill Richardson Drive was part of the street race circuit for the Burt Munro Challenge – an annual meeting made up of several events held over several days. In recent years it had become a mecca for motorcyclists, who rode from all parts of the country to attend the rally. For me, 'The Burt' was my favourite meeting in NZ as you got to race in several different disciplines throughout the week.

The street race was held in a one block, rectangular circuit. A little imagination was put into it with some hay bales which created chicanes down three of the four straights. Street racing, being inherently dangerous, was a hard sell when applying for approval from the authorities. Chicanes were a way of slowing the riders down. Riders didn't want to be slowed down – their bikes had several gears, shame to only use a few of them. However, drop a green flag on them and they would stop bitching and start racing – like their lives depended on it.

The town of Wyndham had been used for street races before the Invercargill event. I had done the Wyndham race once. The Wyndham course was an enclosed square with hay bales on every corner – blocking off any escape route. I described it as 'cage fighting on motorcycles'.

I preferred the Invercargill racetrack and I had done it a few times with varying results. I had come second that very year. I had won it before. I had also crashed there in the rain. And I had blown up a bike while leading the race. Winning, nearly winning, crashing and blowing up: a tidy summary of a racing season.

I always felt at home in Invercargill. Many of its streets were named after rivers in Scotland. The Scottish blood ran strong in Invercargill.

The cycle trail followed the Waihopai River, which became estuary and then harbour. There were a few people using the cycleway – more walkers than cyclists. The cycleway didn't go all the way to Bluff; but it would – it was being worked on and the hope was that it would be completed by the following year. It would be awesome to cycle between Invercargill and Bluff without the fear of being flattened like a pancake.

Highway One to Bluff was notorious for being unpleasant on a bike. The traffic was intense during a working week, with lots of trucks. There was no record of a cyclist being killed on this section of road – there's no 'tales of terror' records kept. I considered myself lucky it was the weekend – only one truck and trailer unit passed me. The driver was very considerate and both slowed and gave me a wide berth. The yin and yang of truck drivers. I had been passed by only two truckies that morning. One an arse. The other a gentleman. I also thought that no matter how bad the traffic could get, it was preferable to being in a sinking fishing boat off Amity.

Hooper had gone down in the shark cage with some misbegotten plan to kill the fish and Jaws went straight through the bars and ate him – quick and simple. In the movie, Hooper survived to swim back to shore – he and Chief Brody amicably using a piece of flotsam. Of course, in the movie Hooper's not having Brody's wife, so it could be amicable.

The road to Bluff made a vast sweep to the left. Many were mistaken into thinking the hill that you saw straight ahead was Bluff Hill. To spot Bluff you needed to swivel your head 90 degrees left, and there it was in the distance. Unmistakeable, if you knew. Thus, much like the end of 90 Mile Beach, it never appeared to be getting closer. The yin and yang of the TA.

Light rain began falling, which seemed fitting. The sky was an oppressively low, slate grey – there was a heaviness to it; it was the bottom of the world. Skipper Quint was being devoured as I went past the large, rusted Bluff sign. I had made Bluff – but, the true ending for the TA was at Stirling Point, beneath the famous signpost.

Rain falling and a flat steel-grey sea greeted me as I passed through the township of Amity – sorry, Bluff. Bluff was named for the brooding hill that loomed over the town.

Bluff Hill was the scene of the shortest motorcycle races I had ever competed in: The Bluff Hillclimb was one part of the Burt Munro. Strangely, it was the hill climb that I loved the most. Bluff Hill had a gradient of 10.7 precent, which in bicycle talk was, 'Feckin Hard'. I had done the race several times but the one that stuck in my brain was in 2015. I had parked my truck for the night on the side street beside the start line. I woke to a murky morning with clouds roiling a chaotic sky. Over a cup of tea I observed, out of the truck window, the organisers trying to manhandle a semblance of order into the general apparatus needed to run a timed race meeting. The wind was roaring and thrashing at them in their yellow PVC gear; there was a reason it was called the Challenge. I enjoyed it immensely. This was what I had driven three days from Whangārei to do. My hardy Celtic genes came alive, and, combined with a certain obtuseness, provided the formula for me to enjoy the going when the going got intense.

I remembered being on the start line. The old fella – who could really tell his age under all that PVC? – put the chock under the back wheel to prevent the bike rolling backwards. The other old fella, pointed at the start lights and pointed to me. He gave me the thumbs up. I returned the sign.

The rain was coming in sheets directly from Foveaux Strait. Seagulls above and forwards of me were trying to make some headway but were being blown backwards. *Concentrate, DC.*

The light went green and it was off. Try not to wheelie too much – although you want to. Short shift to second gear and turn right. Get hard on the gas and head for the spectators huddled on the outside of the next turn. Left here, still on the gas, then brake hard and tip into the right. This is a smooth corner but notoriously slippery. When it's dry there's a spring two-thirds of the way across it to provide a water feature. That day the whole road was awash. On the gas and the rear lets go just enough to check the pucker switch has been engaged. Then its full chat up the short straight and once again aim for the spectators on the outside of the corner. (This was the only course I had raced on where there was no fencing and spectators spread willy-nilly wherever they wanted – including the outside of the corners. My fellow competitors and I were very aware of this, *how could you not be*, and rode within ourselves to reduce the chances of calamitous crashing. The organisers were also very aware of this and limited the number of runs – the racers, as racers do, got faster with each run – corresponding with the raising of the risk factor to friend and foe).

Brake hard but quickly and lay the bike onto its left, but not too much, as the pavement was often unstable and loose here. This was the main straight and the reason I loved the hill climb. Crouch low, lift the bum off the seat, stand on the pegs and nail it. Hold it pinned and shift gears. The tortured engine would scream as the bike leapt, touched down, found air – ripping at the potholes for traction; total concentration – you weren't thinking about your mortgage or what you're having for dinner. Then brake as late as possible for the last right hander – a sweet, sweeping knee down corner. That was it.

I had done 'The Burt' a couple of weeks before starting the TA. I had driven to Bluff for the hill climb with the wind threatening to blow the truck off the road. Torrential rain and 30 knot winds, plus gusts, meant the organisers had to call it quits – for the first time ever.

Bluff's first pub, The Eagle, appeared on my right. The harbour was on the left. I imagined what was just below the surface of those seemingly benign waters. Great Whites were slowly patrolling, their massive tails sweeping side to side. Chief Brody finally dispatched the great fish. It was over. I looked across the gunmetal grey water and felt a bond – the chief and me linked forever, both having completed our missions despite the blood and tears.

The township of Bluff was weatherworn but hardy, as were the nearly 2000 people who lived there. Bluff summers were cool, its winters were short and cold. Rainfall didn't vary much, month to month, but the wind really cranked up from August to December. I wasn't overly appreciative at having to ride the extra three km into the wind just to get my photo taken. However, friends and family had warned me not to return home without a picture.

I cycled over the rise and into Stirling Point. There were a couple of young fellas beside a ute, stripping out of their camo wetsuits. They had spearguns and a few fish lying about.

'That's incredible,' I spluttered, pulling my bike up beside them. 'I'm so glad to see you alive. I just this moment finished the talking book, *Jaws*. And here you are, just come out of the sea. And you're alive.' I gasped expectantly, eyes wide with worry.

The spear fishermen looked at one another and shrugged their shoulders. I looked back and forth at each of them, a loopy grin on my face.

'Okay,' I said, suddenly realising they had no idea what I was on about – or what drugs I was on. 'Good work, men.' I rolled my bike away from them. They probably had no idea what *Jaws* was. I considered: would they have even been born when it came out. Surely everyone knew about *Jaws*?

There were plenty of people milling about at Stirling Point, despite the rain. Getting their pics taken beside the celebrated yellow sign. Cape Reinga 1403km, Equator 5133km, Hobart 1608km, South Pole 4810km, etc.

A young couple had just finished taking each other's photo and were happy to oblige me. I tried to explain to them it was important as I had just cycled from Cape Reinga. They didn't comprehend – they smiled and shook their heads sympathetically, as if expressing concern at the pain I must be going through. Sympathy – perhaps it was the best emotion I could hope for.

Many TA'ers jubilantly lifted their bike overhead to signal their conquest – it did make a great image. I didn't think I could physically do that, and I didn't want to. Luigi had told me that he would lift his bike over his head, 'then throw the bastard into the sea'. I smiled at that image and wondered if he had – Luigi should have finished the day before.

It was wet, cold and a little bleak at the point. Curiously, I was pleased about this. You didn't find a tiki bar and a pina colada waiting at the top of Everest.

The celebration was within – the contented warmth of a job well done. The glow of achievement that, despite the odds, I had overcome them. Fear and loneliness had wanted to become my new constant companions, but I had kept them at bay. Despair and deep confusion had ridden alongside; I had refused them a seat. This was a profound, life-altering moment to be savoured.

I had none of those feelings. In fact, I felt ... nothing. Here I was, stood at the bottom of the mainland of NZ, having cycled 3000 kilometres, but there was no sensation of – anything – nada.

My legs were supremely fit and I had lost five kilos. The trip had taken 33 days, including four rest days. The TA 'rules' were that you should do it in under 30. *Tant pis, to that.* So that was 3000 km divided by 29 ride days.

There would be no more getting up and riding every day for around 10 hours. Cycling had become as automatic as breathing.

'...when a man lets things go so far that he is more than half a bicycle, you will not see him so much because he spends a lot of his time leaning with one elbow on walls or standing propped by one foot at kerbstones.'

Flan O'Brien – The Third Policeman

I was the Lanterne Rouge.

'Well, little buddy,' I said, thoughtfully patting Homer's head. 'We made it. Knocked the bugger off.'

'Yes, we did, partner,' agreed Homer. 'And I can't thank you enough for bringing me on this trip.'

'Don't mention it,' I chuckled.

'No. I can't thank you. Enough. But we did, "knock the bugger off",' chortled Homer.

'What are you going to do now?' I asked.

'I miss Marge. I'm going to head home. And I've got another two seasons of The Simpsons booked.'

'Well, Homer. I've got a room booked at The Eagle. What say we finish this saga with oysters and beer?'

'Mmmn beer.'

'Life is not a journey to the grave with the intention of arriving safely in a well preserved body, but rather to skid in broadside, thoroughly used up, totally worn out, and loudly proclaiming, "Wow what a ride!"'

—HST

Thanks

To my editor Michelle Elvy for putting a head and a tail on it … and calling it a Duck. For teaching me English – and she being American. And for reminding me that Homer is a real person.

www.ingramcontent.com/pod-product-compliance
Lightning Source LLC
Chambersburg PA
CBHW011148290426
44109CB00024B/2534